HOME HEALTH NURSING:
SCOPE AND STANDARDS
OF PRACTICE

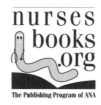

nurses
books
.org

The Publishing Program of ANA

AMERICAN NURSES ASSOCIATION
SILVER SPRING, MARYLAND
2008

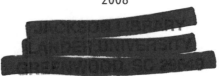

Library of Congress Cataloging-in-Publication data

American Nurses Association.

  Home health nursing : scope and standards of practice. — 2007 rev.
    p. ; cm.
Rev. ed. of: Scope and standards of home health nursing practice. c1999.

  Includes bibliographical references and index.
  ISBN-13: 978-1-55810-255-2 (pbk.)
  ISBN-10: 1-55810-255-8 (pbk.)
  1. Home nursing—Standards—United States.   2. Visiting nurses—Training of—
United States.   I. American Nurses Association. Scope and standards of home health
nursing practice.   II. Title.

[DNLM: 1. Home Care Services—standards—United States. WY 115 A512hm 2007]

RT120.H65A44 2007
610.73'43—dc22   2007037573

The American Nurses Association (ANA) is a national professional association. This ANA publication— *Home Health Nursing: Scope and Standards of Practice*—reflects the thinking of the nursing profession on various issues and should be reviewed in conjunction with state board of nursing policies and practices. State law, rules, and regulations govern the practice of nursing, while *Home Health Nursing: Scope and Standards of Practice* guides nurses in the application of their professional skills and responsibilities.

Published by Nursesbooks.org
The Publishing Program of ANA

American Nurses Association
8515 Georgia Avenue, Suite 400
Silver Spring, MD 20910-3492
1-800-274-4ANA
http://www.nursesbooks.org/

ANA is the only full-service professional organization representing the nation's 2.9 million Registered Nurses through its 54 constituent member associations. ANA advances the nursing profession by fostering high standards of nursing practice, promoting the economic and general welfare of nurses in the workplace, projecting a positive and realistic view of nursing, and lobbying the Congress and regulatory agencies on healthcare issues affecting nurses and the public.

Design: Scott Bell, Arlington, VA; Freedom by Design, Alexandria, VA; Stacy Maguire, Sterling, VA ~ *Editing & indexing*: Steven A. Jent, Denton, TX ~ *Proofreading*: Lisa Munsat Anthony, Chapel Hill, NC ~ *Composition*: House of Equations, Inc., Arden, NC ~ *Printing*: McArdle Printing, Upper Marlboro, MD

First printing October 2007.

ISBN-13: 978-1-55810-255-2   SAN: 851-3481   3M   10/07

ACKNOWLEDGMENTS

The work group that created this 2007 revision of *Home Health Nursing: Scope and Standards of Practice* gratefully acknowledges the work of previous task forces in 1999, 1992, and 1986 to initiate the original documents on home health care.

Work Group Members (2007)

Marilyn D. Harris, MSN, RN, CNAA-BC, FAAN, Chair
Laura Beth Brown, MSN, C, RN
Joann K. Erb, PhD, RN
Soozi Flannigan, MSN, RN, APRN
Lisa A. Gorski, MS, APRN-BC, CRNI, FAAN
Carolyn J. Humphrey, MS, RN, FAAN
Patricia M. Hunt, MS, RN
Deana M. Kilmer, MBA, BS, RN
N. Jean Macdonald, MS, RN
Karen S. Martin, MSN, RN, FAAN
Paula Milone-Nuzzo, PhD, RN, FAAN, FHHC
Mary Narayan, MSN, APRN-BC, CTN
Mary St. Pierre, MSN, RN, MGA
Jeanie Stoker, MPA, RN-BC
Cynthia Struk, PhD, RN, PNP
Denise Swegles, BSN, RN, CHA

ANA Staff

Carol J. Bickford, PhD, RN-BC—Content editor
Patricia Rowell, PhD, APRN-BC—Content editor
Yvonne D. Humes, MSA—Project coordinator
Therese Myers, JD—Legal counsel

Contents

PREFACE

Home Health Nursing: Scope and Standards of Practice describes the professional practice of all home health registered nurses. This scope statement and these updated standards of home health nursing practice are meant to guide, define, and direct home health professional nursing practice.

The American Nurses Association (ANA) has been active in the development of scope of practice and standards since the late 1960s. ANA published the first standards (*Standards of Nursing Practice*) for the nursing profession in 1973 (included in ANA, 2004). These standards were generic in nature and focused on the basic nursing process—a critical thinking model applicable to all registered nurses—composed of assessment, diagnosis, outcomes identification, planning, implementation, and evaluation (ANA, 2005, p.10; ANA, 2004, p. 3). Various revisions have ensued, the most recent being *Nursing: Scope and Standards of Practice* (ANA, 2004), which is to be used in conjunction with *Nursing's Social Policy Statement, 2nd Edition* (ANA, 2003) and *Code of Ethics for Nurses with Interpretive Statements* (ANA, 2001). These three resources provide a complete and definitive description for better understanding of nursing practice and nursing's accountability to the public in the United States (ANA, 2004, p. *vi*).

Specialty nursing organizations have affirmed the 2004 ANA publication by using the template language of the standards when developing scope of practice statements and standards of practice for registered nurses in specialty practice. ANA published the first *Standards of Home Health Nursing Practice* in 1986; a revision followed in 1992. The 1999 revision, *Scope and Standards of Home Health Nursing Practice*, included a scope of practice statement to describe the specialty practice as well as its revised standards of practice. This latest revision (2007) includes a contemporary scope of practice statement and accompanying standards of practice to guide home health nursing practice today and in the future.

As part of its regular process of development, review, and maintenance of scope and standards of nursing practice, ANA convened a volunteer work group of home health nursing professionals in 2005 to review and revise the 1999 standards to best reflect contemporary home health nursing practice and provide a framework for future practice.

Registered nurses in different home health settings and in various roles responded to ANA's call for volunteers. They have worked on the document in small groups and through monthly conference calls since September 2005. The work group:

- assessed research reports, publications, and evidence-based practice;
- distributed and sought input on the updated draft scope and standards from nurses who attended the Home Healthcare Nurses Association (HHNA) meetings at the National Association for Home Care and Hospice (NAHC) annual meetings in October 2005 and 2006;
- shared information and requested input from nurses through a guest editorial in *Home Healthcare Nurse* (Harris, 2006);
- notified ANA's Constituent Member Associations (CMAs), specialty nursing organizations, home health organizations, and other stakeholders that input was requested on the document; and
- posted the draft document on ANA's Web site for public review and comment by interested nurses and others.

All public comments and suggestions were considered by the work group in preparing the final document. Reviews by the Committee on Nursing Practice Standards and Guidelines of the ANA Congress on Nursing Practice and Economics culminated in the final edits, acknowledgment of the scope of practice, approval of the standards of practice, and publication of this, the 2008 updated edition, *Home Health Nursing: Scope and Standards of Practice.*

The profession must incorporate the updated content on these pages into home health nursing practice across the country. The goal is to improve the health, well-being, and quality of life of all home healthcare patients and their families and other caregivers. This can best be accomplished through the significant and visible contributions of registered nurses using standards-based practice.

HOME HEALTH NURSING SCOPE OF PRACTICE

Evolution of Home Health Nursing

The specialty of home health nursing is rapidly growing and evolving because of demographic changes and technological advances. While community-based care has been provided for centuries, Florence Nightingale, William Rathbone, and their colleagues formalized the practice during the 1800s. The titles they selected—district nurses (home health) and health visitors (public health)—are still in use in the United Kingdom.

During the late nineteenth and early twentieth centuries, home health nursing services were organized in many cities and towns in the United States. Frequently, women from wealthy families provided the leadership and resources to establish nursing services. Although few of the women were nurses, they were genuinely concerned about local health and social issues.

Early nurse leaders, including Lillian Wald, Lavinia Dock, Margaret Sanger, and Mary Breckinridge, refined and publicized models of health promotion and disease prevention. In the late 1800s Visiting Nurse Associations (VNAs) and the nursing divisions of governmental health agencies, such as city and county health departments, provided the majority of services. Community health nurses, as generalists, gave nursing care to the sick as well as health promotion services to individuals, families, and communities. Public health principles and practice, and components of family and community care, were integrated into home-based nursing services.

Several key events drove the steady but slow growth of home care in the early 1900s. In 1909, the Metropolitan Life Insurance Company paid for nurses to care for their policyholders in the home. During World War II, as physicians made fewer home visits and focused instead on offices and hospitals, the home care movement grew, with nurses providing most of the health and illness care services in the home. In 1946, Montefiore Hospital in New York City developed a post-hospital acute care program and initiated convalescent home care.

In 1952, the American Nurses Association (ANA) and the National League for Nursing (NLN) became the primary national nursing organizations following the merger and restructuring of other organizations.

The NLN became the primary organization for the home health nursing specialty for the next 30 years.

The Medicare legislation of 1965, which included a home health benefit, increased the reach and visibility of home care and led to its significant growth. Because of the new reimbursement benefits, physicians and hospitals began to discharge patients earlier. New treatments and technology enabled more patients to be treated at home, resulting in increased referrals to existing agencies and the establishment of many new agencies, some affiliated with hospitals and some independent, commercial enterprises. Home health nursing practice emphasized acute care in the home, and some agencies began to offer services 24 hours a day, 7 days a week. In addition, the new legislation prompted organizational mergers, including the establishment of the Visiting Nurse Associations of America (VNAA) and the National Association for Home Care (NAHC) in 1982. These two organizations became the primary specialty organizations for home health nurses and continue to provide strong national leadership.

In the early 1980s diagnosis-related groups (DRGs) were phased in over a four-year period in hospitals nationwide. Implementation of the DRG system resulted in shorter hospital stays and increased use of home care services. Home health nurses were faced with providing highly complex clinical care to patients in their homes.

Responding to the expansion of nursing services provided in the home and the need to formalize this specialty practice, ANA published the first version of its practice standards, *Standards of Home Health Nursing Practice*, in 1986. Revised in 1992, this publication was followed by an expanded *Scope and Standards of Home Health Nursing Practice* in 1999.

At the beginning of the twenty-first century, home health nurses provide skilled care in the home that was not anticipated a few years ago. In addition, as a result of pandemic warnings and natural and man-made disasters, the home and community are increasing in importance as the recommended point of care delivery. In the future, home health nurses may be called upon to coordinate and deliver care unlike ever before.

Definition of Home Health Nursing

Home health nursing is the provision of nursing care to acutely ill, chronically ill, terminally ill, and well patients of all ages in their residences. Home health nursing focuses on health promotion and care of the sick while integrating environmental, psychosocial, economic, cultural, and personal health factors affecting an individual's and family's health status (Humphrey & Milone-Nuzzo, 1996–1999, 2008).

Home health nursing is nursing practice applied to patients of all ages in the patients' residences, which may include private homes, assisted living, or personal care facilities. Although there are multiple ways to describe the recipient of home health care—patient, client, customer, and healthcare consumer—this document uses the term *patient*. Patients and their families and other caregivers are the focus of home health nursing practice. The goal of care is to maintain or improve the quality of life for patients and their families and other caregivers, or to support patients in their transition to end of life. This is accomplished through the initiation, coordination, management, and evaluation of resources needed to promote the patient's optimal level of well-being and function. Nursing activities necessary to achieve this goal may include preventive, maintenance, restorative, and rehabilitative interventions to manage existing health problems and prevent potential problems.

Although the term "home care" is used by many national associations and publications, the professional title of home health nurse is defined and recognized by the nursing profession, other healthcare professionals, and the public. The work group members involved in this scope and standards revision considered the terms "home care nurse" and "home health care nurse" and concluded that the title and tradition of *home health nurse* should be continued.

Distinguishing Characteristics of Home Health Nursing

Home health nursing is a specialized area of community health nursing practice which focuses on individuals in need of care in their homes, their families, and their caregivers. Home health nurses provide care to patients across the life span, from the pre-natal through the post-death periods. Home health nursing stresses the holistic management of personal health practices for the treatment of diseases or disability. Practice embraces primary, secondary, and tertiary prevention; assistance to families with coordination of community resources and health insurance benefits; and delivery of healthcare services in a patient's home, including non-conventional residences.

Home health reflects more than a change in location or acute care delivered in the home. Home health requires a change in the definition and structures of care to reflect a broad array of coordinated services, benefits, and caregivers available to patients experiencing complex problems. Home health nurses, who care for these patients, practice independently and require highly developed skills in assessment and care coordination. Although they practice in collaboration with other healthcare professionals, they most often are the only professionals in the home providing care to the patient. As such, they must be expert in assessment, clinical decision-making, and clinical practice. These skills form the foundation for planning, nursing care interventions, communication with other healthcare providers, and referral to other healthcare settings when appropriate.

Home health patients may require nursing care resources 24 hours a day, 7 days a week. The frequency and duration of these services is dependent upon the home care delivery model and holistic needs of the unit that is the patient and the family and other caregivers, ranging from intermittent visits to full-time extended daily care.

Home health nursing differs from other nursing specialties in the degree of responsibility nurses assume in managing the financial cost of care. Home health nurses work directly with public and private payers and with consumer-directed payment programs. Home health nurses must have advanced knowledge of reimbursement systems to help patients obtain the care they need while containing the cost of care.

The Nursing Process in Home Health Nursing

Home health nurses use the nursing process, the essential methodology by which patient goals are identified and achieved. The nursing process is comprised of assessment, diagnosis, outcomes identification, planning, implementation, and evaluation.

Assessment

Home health nurses assess the physical, psychosocial, and environmental factors that affect a patient's health to develop a comprehensive nursing care plan which will attain the patient's desired health outcomes in a culturally comfortable way. Physical assessment includes systems assessment, impact of the disease or condition on the patient, and monitoring of medications and therapies. Psychosocial assessment includes family, cultural, and spiritual assessments. Environmental assessment includes assessing the patient's safety, ability to meet daily needs, and ability to participate in meaningful activities in the home. In the home setting, understanding the influences of family dynamics and the home environment on the physical and emotional state of the patient is essential for effective care management.

Diagnosis

Home health nurses derive their diagnoses from the assessment data. Diagnoses can be focused on the physical, psychosocial, cultural, spiritual, environmental, economic, and interpersonal aspects of care. Home health nurses, in collaboration with the patient, the family, and other caregivers, identify actual nursing problems as well as situations that might become problems if unattended. Diagnoses may be specific to nursing practice or may require the home health nurse to serve as a care manager with other members of the interdisciplinary care team.

Outcomes Identification

The home health nurse works with the patient, the family, and other caregivers to identify attainable and measurable goals for the patient based on the patient's medical and nursing diagnoses. These goals are the patient outcomes expected as a result of the care the home health nurse and the interdisciplinary team provide. Optimal health and well-being, effective self-management of health problems, or a peaceful death are examples of expected outcomes.

Planning

Home health nurses plan care in collaboration with the patient, family and other caregivers, and other healthcare providers, to develop interventions that are incorporated in the patient's care plan. When the patient receives services from multiple practitioners, including non-professionals, home health nurses often assume the role of care manager and coordinate all the involved disciplines, including the patient's primary care provider and other caregivers, to optimize patient outcomes.

The home health nurse provides clinical supervision to Licensed Practical/Vocational Nurses (LPN/LVN) and home health aides in accordance with the Medicare Conditions of Participation (COPs) and state practice standards. According to a 2002 study (Stoker, 2003), all 50 states allow LPN/LVNs to provide home care under the direct and indirect supervision of an RN. As a home health nurse, the RN must be aware of the responsibility in the supervision and delegation processes as defined by the profession, state practice acts, accrediting bodies, and agency policy.

Implementation

Home health nurses provide skilled nursing interventions to patients and their families and caregivers, including teaching, counseling, care management, resource coordination, and evaluative data collection. In collaboration with the patient, the family, and other caregivers, home health nurses determine the most appropriate nursing care strategies to meet identified patient outcomes, which often include complementary and cultural therapies.

Patient and family and other caregiver teaching is integral to the role of home health nurses. Teaching supports the achievement of patient outcomes and the movement of the patient and the family toward independence. As expert patient educators, home health nurses use a variety of media and strategies to develop and reinforce enhanced self-care skills. Home health nurses share knowledge of community health resources with the patient, the family, and other caregivers. Through this information exchange and advocacy, home health nurses encourage patients, families, and other caregivers to plan for and seek additional services as their needs dictate.

One of the primary responsibilities of home health nurses is patient advocacy. This is incorporated in all phases of the nursing process, not just during implementation of the plan of care and associated therapies. Patient advocacy includes assisting patients in navigating the healthcare delivery system, supporting them in making healthcare decisions, and helping them access community resources to support independence. Informing, supporting, and affirming that the decision-making of patients, their families, and other caregivers are important adjuncts to achieving patient care objectives and patient goals.

The home health nurse will also assess the implementation of the care plan and care provided by the LPN/LVN and home health aide. While the LPN/LVN and home health aide may be team members in the home health setting, the RN must provide ongoing assessment and supervision as required by the law to help ensure positive outcomes.

Home health nursing is provided in the context of a highly differentiated and complex healthcare delivery system and requires special time management and organizational skills. To help patients achieve desired health outcomes, home health nurses need specific knowledge about the dynamic financial and regulatory aspects of care that are unique to this practice.

Evaluation

The evaluation of patient outcomes provides critical data to determine the effectiveness of nursing care. Home health nurses must critically evaluate their practice through quality improvement activities, critical incident reviews, and participation in research.

Educational Preparation of Home Health Nurses

Home health nursing, because of its level of independence in practice, requires a high degree of knowledge and expertise. Although baccalaureate nurses are better prepared to meet the demands of home health nursing practice, nurses with associate degrees or diplomas can enter home health nursing as members of the nursing team. All nurses who enter home health nursing are expected to grow in their ability to assume home health nursing's roles and demands through the support of their colleagues, structured preceptor programs, clinical experiences, and lifelong learning through academic and continuing education. At this time certification as a home health nurse is not available. However, home health nurses can affirm their knowledge and skills through other applicable nursing certification in such areas as pediatrics, critical care, hospice and palliative care, and gerontological nursing.

Home Health Nurse: Generalist

Home health nurses provide all aspects of nursing care in accord with *Nursing: Scope and Standards of Practice* (ANA, 2004), as well as the more detailed home health nursing standards. Competent home health nursing practice requires flexibility, creativity, and innovative approaches to situations and problems in the context of individual and environmental differences and widely varying resource availability.

Effective home health nursing practice includes identification of and attention to environmental, economic, familial, and cultural differences. In addition, a basic understanding of psychosocial and safety issues affecting patients, their families, and other caregivers is critical for the effective delivery of home health nursing. Because patients residing in their homes may receive healthcare services from an array of providers, home health nurses must assume the role of care manager and coordinator.

Therefore, the preferred minimum qualifications for a registered nurse practicing in the home health setting are:

- A baccalaureate degree in nursing.
- Ability to incorporate communication and motivation skills and principles in the home health setting.
- Ability to apply critical thinking to physical, psychosocial, environmental, cultural, family, and safety issues.
- Ability to utilize clinical decision-making in applying the nursing process to patients in their places of residence.
- Ability to practice as an effective member of an interdisciplinary team.
- Competency in applying care management skills.

Home health nursing is an autonomous practice requiring knowledge and skills often not attained in basic nursing educational programs or other practice settings. Therefore, all registered nurses (RN) must be initially assessed for their ability to apply the nursing process to the home health setting, including consideration of prior home care and general nursing practice experience and educational preparation.

The necessary knowledge base and skills for home health nursing can be developed through formal orientation programs, structured preceptor programs, and guided clinical experience based on the specific learning needs of the nurse. Each home health nurse must build and maintain the professional knowledge, skills, and abilities that support evidence-based practice and clinical decision-making that empowers the patient to attain self-management and achieve the best outcomes possible. The employing agency also has an obligation to establish an environment conducive to such professional development.

Home Health Nurse: Advanced Practice

Advanced practice registered nurses (APRN) working in home health settings possess advanced specialized clinical knowledge and skills to provide health care to patients, families, and groups in their places of residence. The Clinical Nurse Specialist (CNS) and Nurse Practitioner (NP) are the advanced practice RNs who most frequently practice in home health.

The increasingly older and chronically ill home health patient population requires a high level of clinical expertise as treatment and medication regimens have grown in complexity. These patient characteristics, combined with the pressure to improve clinical outcomes, require more advanced practice nurses in home health.

Advanced practice registered nurses hold a master's or doctoral degree in nursing. They build on the practice of registered nurses by demonstrating a greater depth and breadth of knowledge, a greater synthesis of data, increased complexity of skills and interventions, and significant role autonomy (ANA, 2004, p.14). The APRN in home health settings evaluates and implements evidence-based practice to improve care for patients and families, develops specialized programs that promote improvement in clinical outcomes, collaborates with community resources, and may participate in research pertaining to home health nursing practice and home health services.

APRNs may prescribe pharmacologic and non-pharmacologic treatments in the direct management of acute and chronic illness and disease in compliance with federal and state regulations in the home health setting. APRNs are specially suited to the development and management of outcomes-based research in the area of home care. The APRN may also assume the role of nurse educator and mentor undergraduate nursing students and graduate level practitioners in home health practice.

Clinical Nurse Specialist

The CNS is an expert in evidence-based nursing practice, treating and managing the health concerns of patients, families, and populations. CNS practice is targeted toward achieving quality, cost-effective outcomes in accordance with three spheres of influence (NACNS, 2004):

- *Patient care* –Comprehensive assessment, expert care and care planning, care management for home health patients, families, and groups with specific or complex needs, and application of evidence-based clinical interventions for patient populations with similar needs or disease states.

- *Nurses and nursing practice* – Meeting the educational needs of nurses through formal and informal methods, promoting evidence-based practice to achieve clinical outcomes, acting as a consultant to staff and administration in the area of improving clinical outcomes.

- *Organization or system* – Initiating change and continuous improvement to benefit the system, developing and implementing evidence-based, best practice models, development of programs for groups of patients that enhance patient outcomes.

Nurse Practitioner

Nurse practitioners (NPs) perform comprehensive assessments, diagnose and treat actual and potential health problems, manage acute and chronic illness, and promote health and the prevention of illness and injury. They diagnose, develop differential diagnoses, and conduct, supervise, and interpret diagnostic and laboratory tests. NPs oversee, manage care, and direct the delivery of clinical services within an integrated system of health care using the transitional and palliative care approaches, thus allowing for continuity of care to and from all settings (home, institution, and community). NPs practice autonomously and in collaboration with other healthcare professionals to treat and manage patients' health problems, and serve as researchers, consultants, and patient advocates for individuals, families, groups, and communities. NPs expand access to services and improve quality of care for patients with advanced chronic illness while improving cost effectiveness.

Roles of the Home Health Nurse

The home health nursing roles detailed below cover: care management and coordination of care, education, advocacy, administration, supervision, and quality improvement.

Care Manager and Coordinator of Care

This role involves not only the delivery of direct care to the patient but also coordination of care provided by other disciplines. When a patient is admitted to service, the nurse care manager uses the nursing process to assess the patient's unique situation, and develops a Plan of Care (POC) in consultation with the patient and the physician. The home health nurse implements the POC to help the patient reach maximal potential and evaluates the outcomes. Specific activities in this process include:

- Performs a comprehensive holistic assessment using the patient, family and other caregivers, and other pertinent sources of information about the patient.

- Designs the POC considering the patient's unique strengths and limitations, and the impact of cultural and religious beliefs on the patient's cognitive, physical, and emotional condition.

- Prioritizes care based on mutual goal setting and outcome identification by the patient and the nurse.

- Provides accurate documentation to support initiation and continuation of skilled services.

- Provides direct care to patients including ongoing assessment of condition, education of the patient and the family, evaluation of effectiveness of care, and revision of POC to achieve the patient's optimal health potential.

- Delegates care to nurses, nursing students, licensed practical nurses (LPNs), and home health aides (HHAs) utilizing the principles of delegation. Provides ongoing instruction and supervision.

- Determines the appropriate utilization of services, acknowledging financial parameters, while developing and implementing a POC that promotes optimal patient outcomes.

- Evaluates the effectiveness of care and the progress of the patient toward goals and revises the plan as needed to help the patient achieve maximal potential and positive outcomes, which may include dying with dignity.

- Collaborates with the interdisciplinary team and maintains communication related to the patient's response to the POC.

- Collaborates with the healthcare providers by communicating changes in condition and progress toward goal attainment.

Educator

Home health nurses educate patients, families and other caregivers, and the community. A major responsibility of home health nurses is to provide instruction to patients, families, and other caregivers on acute and chronic disease processes, and to help patients develop other self-management skills and abilities. In this role, nurses provide information, demonstrate techniques, and evaluate performance of procedures by patients, families, and other caregivers. Nurses must be able to identify barriers to learning, provide instructions using a variety of methods, and incorporate health beliefs and cultural and religious practices into the process of patient education. The home health nurse also:

- Educates patients, families, and other caregivers on healthy lifestyle, health promotion, and disease prevention.

- Provides information and education concerning reimbursement for home care services.

Nurses may also conduct community education programs and provide information about available home health services and reimbursement for care. Home health nurses educate physicians and other health professionals about opportunities to work collaboratively in the home setting. The goals for collaboration include helping the patient achieve optimal function, maintain independence, and in some cases helping terminally ill patients remain at home.

Advocate

The home health nurse is often the health professional who interacts most with patients, their families, and other caregivers. As a result of this interaction, nurses frequently become aware of problems or circumstances that interfere with a patient's recovery, safety, or well-being. Home health nurses treat the individual in a holistic manner and recognize when additional clarification or support is needed or additional resources are required. Nurses may also identify factors that interfere with a patient's recovery, safety, or adherence to the treatment plan. As advocates, home health nurses serve as a liaison between the patient, the family (as providers of care), healthcare provider, and the healthcare system; provide information to assist in informed decision-making; and support decisions that a patient makes. The home health nurse also:

- Identifies and coordinates community resources to assist patients in achieving maximum health potential.
- Empowers patients and families in their interactions with the health-care system by providing information and support.
- Provides information about care options, reimbursement, and community resources.
- Implements programs, such as medication reconciliation and fall prevention, to maximize patient safety.
- Refers the patient to community services and resources to ensure continuity of care after discharge from home care.
- Promotes continuity of care through collaboration within the agency and with other healthcare providers.

The home health nurse is also accountable for advocacy for both professional development and the professional practice of home health nursing. The responsibilities include ongoing education, mentoring, contributing to the ongoing development of the practice through active participation in professional membership, promoting the image of professional home health nursing, and actively participating in legislation and research that affect home health nursing. Other professional advocacy responsibilities include:

- Acting as a role model for professional nursing and as a proactive nursing advocate.
- Supporting and encouraging others to study and practice nursing.
- Sharing knowledge and experience with colleagues within and outside of home health.
- Serving as a leader in health promotion and patient care by advancing one's own knowledge base.
- Incorporating concepts of evidence-based practice in planning nursing interventions.
- Fostering cohesive relationships and collaborating with all members of the nursing profession.

- Maintaining membership and active involvement in professional organizations to remain current in health policy that impacts practice.
- Participating in formal quality assessment and improvement activities.

Administrator

The home health administrator is responsible for maintaining quality care in a dynamic environment in which reimbursement requirements, accreditation standards, and healthcare systems change frequently. The administrator provides leadership to meet these challenges and ensure availability of competent, qualified staff. The administrator must be knowledgeable about computerization, financial issues, documentation, and new opportunities while maintaining organizational and patient care standards. As the conscience of the organization, the administrator concentrates on the mission of the organization and its first priority, namely the patient and the patient's needs. The administrator also serves as a liaison between staff and outside agencies, including national and legal entities. The administrator speaks for home health staff and patients and brings attention to problems and limitations of the present system.

Supervisor

The home health supervisor, or clinical manager, is responsible for the coordination and evaluation of patient care activities. The supervisor facilitates the professional development of home health nurses by providing education and support in clinical decision-making, disease management, and compliance with regulations related to home health services. The supervisor supports achievement of the organization's mission and goals by ensuring the availability of a competent nursing staff.

Quality Improvement Expert

The nurse leader who is responsible for quality improvement promotes excellence in clinical practice in the organization. This includes the collection and analysis of quantitative and qualitative data to evaluate patients' responses to care. The nurse evaluates the organization's processes and structure to ensure quality care and incorporates scientific evidence into policies, procedures, and practices. The nurse also provides education and support and may mentor new staff or supervisors. This role includes translating and disseminating quality data to appropriate stakeholders.

Trends, Issues, and Opportunities

Home health nurses, their organizations, and the healthcare industry face exciting, although sobering, trends, issues, and opportunities. Woven throughout this section are comments about the need for home health nurses and their organizations to:

- Acknowledge the development of health consumerism and increased partnerships with individuals, families, and communities.
- Recognize changing demographics related to aging, chronic illness, and cultural diversity.
- Collaborate with other healthcare professionals and providers.
- Become active change agents rather than reactive participants.
- Note the dramatic impacts of globalization.
- Prepare for the future.

Trends, issues, and opportunities influence the role of today's home health nurse and are likely to do so even more during the next 10 to 20 years.

Practice Issues

Clinical Concerns

Medicare remains the largest single payer of home care: 69% of home care patients are over 65 years old (NAHC, 2004). Chronic illnesses are increasingly common among older adults and account for the majority of home health diagnoses. Chronic illnesses are also costly, accounting for more than 70% of the cost of health care in the United States each year (CDC, 2004). Chronically ill patients frequently require multiple medications, ongoing treatment, and monitoring. The impact on quality of life and functional ability is significant. Many patients with chronic illnesses that require lifestyle modification as part of their care plan do not adhere to such recommendations to manage their illnesses. With an increasing emphasis on healthcare outcomes, home health nurses are challenged to work more effectively with the chronically ill.

The World Health Organization (2003) emphasizes that working with patients to improve adherence to treatment and medication protocols is of critical importance to patient safety, overall health, and reducing the cost of health care. Home health nurses must rise to the challenge of identifying barriers to adherence and helping patients self-manage their illnesses. Home health nurses must work collaboratively with patients and families to set realistic healthcare goals, adopt problem-solving skills, manage symptoms, and reduce the risk for disease exacerbation.

Home health clinical practice continues to include care of acutely ill patients, allowing for early discharge of hospitalized patients to receive more complex treatments such as advanced wound care treatments and infusion therapies at home. With improved drug therapies and home monitoring capabilities, some patients with diagnoses such as infections and deep vein thrombosis can be treated at home without hospitalization. When managing acute conditions in the home setting, the safety of the home environment is essential in relation to both the types of treatments provided and the presence of caregiver support.

While home health nurses must function as generalists caring for a wide variety of patients and conditions, increasingly there will be an emphasis on specialty areas of expertise. For example, there is growing interest in providing palliative care and behavioral health programs in the home health environment. Home health programs for prevalent diagnoses such as heart failure or diabetes, promotion of specialized home health nursing skills, and use of advanced practice nurses are increasingly cited as effective home health strategies associated with improved clinical outcomes.

For home health nurses, one goal has always been to help patients remain healthy and avoid acute care hospitalization. This outcome has become a focus of national concern as hospitalization contributes to the ever increasing risk and cost of health care. In a recent study, a number of strategies were identified as important to reducing hospitalization among home health patients including clinical strategies of preventing falls, medication management, case management, patient and caregiver education, and disease management programs (NAHC, 2006).

Home health agencies are responding to an environment of consumerism by better defining their services and developing new services to meet the needs of the community and healthcare payers. This consumer focus helps ensure that home health services promote wellness, especially among high-risk patients living in the community. Examples include fall prevention, medication safety, pain management, education related to infection prevention, and immunization programs.

The ability to measure and compare outcomes using Outcome Assessment and Information Set (OASIS) data has had a major impact on home health nursing. As home health evolves into a pay-for-performance model of reimbursement, home health nurses will become better educated about and accountable to achieving positive patient outcomes. Home health nurses must use effective strategies to provide home health care with attention to age and developmental stages, cultural issues, and evidence-based practices.

The steep increase in the older adult population, the rising prevalence of chronic illnesses, and the challenges of cultural diversity will significantly affect home health practice in the future. Home health services will become an even more critical element of the healthcare system by controlling the overall cost of healthcare, keeping patients out of expensive acute care hospitals, and reducing the need for patients to reside in long-term care facilities.

Ethics

In the general world of health care, the patient is the "outsider" and is expected to behave according to the "rules" of the hospital, outpatient setting, or physician office. Home health care is unique because the home health nurse is the "outsider" with the patient, family, and other caregivers "allowing" the nurse to provide care in their home. Home health nurses provide care in settings ranging from the most luxurious mansions to tents under a bridge. They recognize that patients' homes are their "castles" and the optimal places to educate and promote health.

Home health nurses may face numerous ethical issues during the course of care. The patient's privacy may be compromised as family members and caregivers are taught to provide care. Patients or family members or caregivers may fail to comply with healthcare recommendations such as treatments or medications. Care provided by family members or caregivers may be poor, even neglectful or abusive. Patients may choose to follow medical, nutritional, pharmacological, and other courses that are not within the plan of care or optimal to their health. Patients may require services beyond what the home health agency is able to provide or beyond what the insurance or other payer will cover. Physicians may order treatments that conflict with best practice. Challenges arise when home health nurses must balance patient needs with personal safety, such as animals or illegal activities in the home.

Home health nurses must explore their own personal values in relation to the rules and regulations that influence practice. *Code of Ethics for Nurses with Interpretive Statements* (ANA, 2001) provides guidance. The home health nurse acts as a patient advocate and maintains confidentiality, safety, security, dignity, and respect for both the patient and the family. Home health agencies must provide guidelines and resources for ethical issues that arise. Increasingly, home health agencies utilize interdisciplinary ethics committees to explore ethical issues and formulate plans to resolve such issues.

Legislation, Regulations, Legal Obligations, and Licensure

"Government's influence on professional practice, quality health care, and agency administration increases with each passing year. Federal, state, and local laws and regulations impact the day-to-day operations." (Mebus & Piskor, 2005, p. 675). It is important for home health nurses to understand how they can influence the legislative and regulatory processes, identify resources, and take action when necessary. Furthermore, they must be knowledgeable about and comply with existing statutes and regulations. Information about legislation, regulations, and legal matters is available from government agencies, such as the Centers for Medicare and Medicaid Services and state and local health departments, in government publications like the *Federal Register*, and through employers and professional and trade associations.

Legislation

Home health nurses have a responsibility to be aware of and seek to influence federal, state, and local legislation that affects the nursing profession. In addition, home health nurses should actively work to influence legislation that affects the delivery of healthcare services in the home. These goals can be accomplished by monitoring professional and trade associations for information about congressional activities and state and local legislative initiatives, and by taking action to influence legislation through advocacy. Formal organizations, such as professional and trade associations, provide a variety of venues for legislative action.

Regulations

Home health nurses must be knowledgeable of federal, state, and local regulations that govern their practice, including nurse licensure requirements. In addition, they should be knowledgeable of and adhere to federal, state, and local quality, payment, and general health and hygiene regulations, and safe work practices. Ideally, home health nurses should participate in the regulatory process by taking an active role in such activities as government technical expert panels and submission of formal comments on proposed regulations.

Legal Obligations and Licensure

Legal obligations of home health nurses include compliance with existing statutes and regulations and avoidance of negligence and breach of contract. Legal requirements protect the rights of individuals, ensure fair business practices, impose a legal duty of care, and control fraudulent and abusive practices. The first step in meeting legal obligations is to have an adequate knowledge base. Therefore, home health nurses must first be familiar with federal, state, and local laws.

Home health nurses must adhere to individual professional licensure rules and organizational policies and procedures, which serve as the basis for standards for quantity and quality of care, breach of contract, and patient abandonment. They must know the content of the nurse practice acts for their work settings and understand the implications of the mutual recognition model of nurse licensure if it is applicable. Other patient-centered legal requirements that home health nurses must adhere to include federal, state, and local requirements for privacy and security of health information, civil rights, and the protection of individuals against abuse, neglect, and exploitation. In addition, home health nurses must comply with both state and federal false claims, anti-kickback, and physician self-referral laws and support their employers' compliance efforts. Failure to adhere to legal requirements can result in a wide range of penalties, ranging from disciplinary action against a nursing license and financial liability to criminal charges and exclusion from government programs.

The Nursing Shortage

In 2002 the Joint Commission (formerly the Joint Commission on Accreditation of Healthcare Organizations) reported over 126,000 nursing openings; some home health agencies were being forced to refuse new patients because of a shortfall in home health nurses (Huston, 2006). The gap between the demand for nurses and the supply will continue to grow exponentially. In fact, registered nurses are projected to compose the second largest number of new jobs among all occupations. Home healthcare employment is expected to increase rapidly because of the growing number of older persons with functional disabilities, consumer preference for care in the home, and technological advances that make it possible to bring increasingly complex treatments into the home. (U.S. Department of Labor and Statistics, 2006).

A recent study (Flynn, 2005) examined the factors that attract nurses to and that dissatify them in home health care. The factors that attract included practice flexibility, independence, and more time for direct patient contact that enabled the nurse to teach patients and families (Flynn, 2005). Paperwork and excessive documentation caused the most dissatisfaction; other common issues included overtime work, low salaries, weather, and wear and tear on the car. The increasing cost of transportation affects the entire country and is likely to further impede home health nursing recruitment and retention. Home health administrators are challenged to examine workplace issues such as personal safety and environment, and work with staff to make improvements needed to create attractive employment settings.

Standardized Terminologies and Outcomes Management

Standardized terminologies and outcomes management are mentioned regularly by the public media and payers and are included in most health-related publications and national and international conferences. These factors have an increasingly visible impact on practice, documentation, information management, and reimbursement of home health nurses, their agencies, and the healthcare industry. What works best?

Have patients improved? By how much? From what perspective? How much will it cost? According to Lang, "If we cannot name it, we cannot control it, finance it, teach it, research it, or put it into public policy" (Clark & Lang, 1992).

These questions and the attempts to provide answers are not new. In 1893, physician Jacques Bertillon led an international effort to create a system for statistically classifying the causes of death and disease. Adopted worldwide within a decade, this system led directly to the International Classification of Diseases (ICD) and a series of reference works still in use. The current tenth revision (ICD-10) is used by all member states of the World Health Organization (WHO, 2007). Florence Nightingale was the first nurse to consistently use the scientific method and to transform data into information. In the 1850s she gathered systematic data, transformed a hospital into an efficient institution within 2 months, documented evidence graphically, and publicized her results widely.

During the 1950s and 1960s, nursing leaders in the United States began to conduct evaluation research, explore the relationship of services to client outcomes, and focus on problems that arise with clients out of nursing diagnosis. Simultaneously, physicians advanced systems for nomenclature and classification, including the initial version of Systematized Nomenclature of Medicine (SNOMED). The First National Conference on Classification of Nursing Diagnoses was held in 1973, the same time that the Visiting Nurse Association of Omaha (Nebraska) began to standardize terms for client problems.

In 1989 ANA anticipated outcome management and electronic health record developments that would require standardized terminologies and databases and formed a committee to address these trends. In 1992, the committee recognized four interface terminologies that met selection criteria: NANDA (North American Nursing Diagnosis Association), Omaha System, Home Health Care Classification (HHCC), and Nursing Interventions Classification (NIC). Development and refinement have continued within nursing and other healthcare professions. A total of twelve terminologies and data element sets are currently recognized (ANA, 2006). The additional eight are: International Classification of Nursing Practice (ICNP); Nursing Outcomes Classification (NOC); Perioperative Nursing Data Set; Nursing Minimum Data Set; Nursing Management Minimum Data Set; ABC Codes; Logical Observation Identifiers, Names, and Codes (LOINC®); and SNOMED CT®. Many vendors are adding these terminologies to their software; some are evident to clinician users and others are not visible, such as reference terminologies.

Beginning in 1999, Medicare-certified home health agencies were required to use the Outcome and Assessment Information Set (OASIS), a nationwide attempt to quantify and track patient outcomes of care. Clinicians typically complete this assessment tool of more than 80 items for new patients admitted to home health services. Children and pregnant women are excluded. OASIS data must also be submitted at designated interim periods and at discharge from the home health agency.

Home health agencies participate in outcome-based quality improvement and related quality improvement and benchmarking activities. The Centers for Medicare and Medicaid Services (Centers) publish aggregate clinical data. The Centers indicate they will initiate a new program, "Pay for Performance," that will offer financial incentives for exceeding certain outcome levels and financial penalties for underachievement. Regardless of what the Centers introduces, third-party payers, accreditation and certification groups, private foundations, international governments, and consumers are applying increased pressure on healthcare providers to focus on standardization and outcomes management. Comparison of home health patients, nurses and their professional colleagues, and agencies is the present and the future.

Information Technology and Telehealth

Historically, home health nurses, their clinician colleagues, and their agencies have been innovators and early adopters of communication devices and technology (Rogers, 1995). Clinicians now consider cellular phones a necessity for organizing their schedules, contacting referral sources, and reporting visit findings. Nurses, their agencies, and their patients are now embracing computers, the Internet, and telehealth.

Few home health nurses used telehealth or personal computers in the 1990s because few vendors offered products designed for clinical use. The Internet was launched in 1992. Since 2000, personal, home health agency, and patient use of automation, the Internet, and telehealth have exploded nationally and globally. Many patients and their families use the Internet to become well informed about diagnoses, medications, and treatment. Changes in Medicare regulations and reimbursement have encouraged agencies to invest in hardware and software. Increasingly, home health clinicians complete most of their documentation online for patients' electronic health records.

Many home health agencies have robust clinical, financial, scheduling, and statistical management information systems that are more user-friendly and integrated than their local hospitals' (Martin, 2005). An increasing number of home health agencies use telehealth. Huston (2006) states that as many as 45% of all home health episodes of care may be suitable for telehealth intervention. To understand the application of telehealth to home health nursing, it is important to define it. In its 2001 Report to Congress, the Department of Health and Human Services (2002) defined telehealth as the "use of telecommunication and information technologies to provide healthcare services at a distance to include diagnosis, treatment, public health, consumer health information, and health professions education." A more recent expanded definition (Brantley, Laney-Cummings, & Spivack, 2004) includes the integration of various applications such as clinical health delivery, management of healthcare information, education, and administrative services within a common infrastructure.

Telehealth within the framework of home health nursing can be broadly defined as the delivery of patient care services using technology to eliminate distance, time, or resource barriers in an effort to improve patient health outcomes. Technology applications include but are not limited to the following:

- Telemonitors with peripheral biometric attachments for remotely monitoring biophysical parameters such as weight or more complex measurement such as oxygen saturation or glucose levels.

- Phone technology with two-way connectivity which allows for monitoring of patient activity or response to disease management parameters such as pain, activity level, symptom exacerbation, diet, or behavioral cues. This information may be correlated with biophysical parameters.

- In-home message devices with disease management education, advice, and medication or treatment reminders with compliance monitoring features that may be remotely transmitted via phone or Internet technology or evaluated at nursing visits.

- Video cameras for monitoring all aspects of care delivery particularly focusing on wound management, home care aide supervision, or other aspects of clinical care usually necessitating direct observation.

- Personal computers with Internet connectivity for supervised communication, medical record access, or patient education.

- Video conferencing that allows nurses, physicians, and other healthcare providers to communicate about patient-specific care or to learn new disease management interventions.

Information technology and telehealth can lead to more effective and efficient communication that, in turn, can lead to enhanced quality of care, improved patient and clinician safety, and increased productivity. However, information technology and telehealth cannot replace the necessity or value of direct care. New technology does introduce tension in the workplace and may be threatening because it often represents a significant change, and requires education, financial resources, and new styles of operation (Bowles & Baugh, 2007).

The changes in information technology are dramatic and rapid at all levels in this country and globally. The changes will increasingly influence the practice of home health nurses. The federal government has established the Office of the National Coordinator for Health Information Technology (http://www.hhs.gov/healthit), whose agenda proposes that all documentation be converted to electronic systems in the near future. In addition to providers' electronic health records (EHR; see below), individuals could have microchips to store their own personal health data. Personal EHRs may become the norm rather than the exception in the near future.

The *electronic health record* is the longitudinal collection of a patient's personal and medical information stored in a computer-readable format. While it has been reported that less than 10% of hospitals in the United States have implemented their technology to include the EHR, home health agencies appear to be utilizing and embracing it. Since 2000, 63% of home health agencies have implemented some type of point-of-care technology (Utterback & Waldo, 2005) that includes various software, hardware, and EHR processes.

SNOMED CT®, LOINC®, and HL7 have been selected as the national standards for providers to link and exchange clinical data. While the governments of the United States and the United Kingdom initially agreed to mandate SNOMED CT, numerous other countries are joining the initiative. Individuals, groups, and countries with the most economic resources are not alone in the use of the Internet and information technology to obtain and communicate health-related information; it is ubiquitous. The regional health information organization (RHIO) effort is intended to encourage collaboration throughout the United States. Vendors are developing and producing smaller and faster digital and multifunctional devices. Web access is expected to replace current technology, and Web-based education is ubiquitous. Today's home health nurses will soon need to use new devices and methods that have not yet been invented. Home health nurses who anticipate and embrace technological developments have evidenced many positive outcomes for their patients.

Research

Diverse research that is pertinent to home health nursing practice includes single studies, studies conducted by members of other disciplines or interdisciplinary teams involving home health nurses, and programs of research. Schumacher and Marren (2004) note the increasing diversity, sophistication, and number of studies published in their extensive literature review. They group their review into five broad areas: nursing classification studies, critical transitions in the illness trajectory, family education and support, specific conditions prevalent in home care, and population diversity. Research priorities identified by Madigan and Vanderboom (2005) include outcomes, health policy, the use of advanced practice nurses, and models of care and best practice.

In general, the number of home health nurse researchers and the extent of funded home health studies are limited, especially in comparison to acute and long-term care research. However, the Centers for Medicare and Medicaid Services (CMS) has identified the reduction of the hospitalization rate of home health patients as a national priority. This emphasis has stimulated research on patient risk factors related to home care and interventions and strategies to reduce risk. A study of home health agencies with the lowest hospitalization rates was recently completed (NAHC, 2006). Fifteen agency strategies were identified as instrumental in preventing hospitalizations; these strategies included assessing and reducing the risks for falls, increasing home visit frequency at the start of care, and giving attention to organizational culture.

Evidence-based practice and evidence-based guidelines are important to home health nurses. Clinical practice guidelines developed by the University of Iowa School of Nursing (e.g., gerontological interventions) and the American Heart Association/American College of Cardiology (e.g., guidelines for heart failure management) are examples of such efforts. While the number of studies specific to home health and capable of serving as a foundation for evidence-based practice is still small, increasing interest will encourage expansion of the research base, increased opportunities for home health nurse researchers, more interdisciplinary collaboration, improved funding, and better client outcomes.

Programs of clinical and administrative research offer the greatest opportunities for continuation and expansion. The following are examples of ongoing research programs that reflect the chronology of evidence-based research and best practices in home health.

- *Omaha System* – The Omaha System is one of the twelve classification systems or standardized terminologies recognized by ANA. Four federally funded studies were conducted between 1975 and 1993 to develop and refine the Omaha System and to establish reliability, validity, and usability. Since then, more than 50 unique studies have been conducted by clinicians, managers, educators, students, and researchers; the studies were organized into eight categories and summarized (Martin, 2005; Monsen & Kerr, 2004; Omaha System, 2006). Most have been published in journals, books, or online.

- *Transitional care* – In the 1980s, Brooten and her colleagues compared outcomes and costs when very low birth weight infants remained hospitalized or were cared for at home by advanced practice nurses, and then expanded their studies to include women and elders (Brooten, et al., 2002 & 2003). McCorkle evolved her symptom distress research to include end-of-life and oncology concerns as well as caregivers' psychosocial status (Jepson et al., 1999; Walke et al., 2006). In 1989, Naylor and Bowles began to study high-risk elders and the discharge planning process (Bowles, 2000; Naylor et al., 2005).

- *Visiting Nurse Service (VNS) of New York* – The VNS of New York established a home health research center in 1994. Its sound research and practice improvement initiative has enabled it to attract major grants from private philanthropies and government funding agencies and increasingly to work collaboratively with the home care industry, academic institutions, and quality improvement organizations to improve geriatric care. The center's initiatives focus on three main areas: improving the quality, cost-effectiveness, and outcomes of home health services; analyzing and influencing public policies that affect home-based care; and supporting communities that promote successful aging in place (Feldman et al., 2004 and 2005; McDonald et al., 2005; Murtaugh et al., 2005).

- *Outcome and Assessment Information Set (OASIS)* – OASIS data are used for home health regulation, reimbursement, clinical purposes, and increasingly in research. Studies have examined inter-rater reliability and accuracy of OASIS (Madigan & Fortinsky, 2004; Madigan, Tullai-McGuinness, & Fortinsky, 2003). OASIS data have been used to analyze and evaluate home health clinical outcomes including outcomes for wound healing and home health service use and adverse events among home health patients (Madigan, 2001; Madigan & Tullai-McGuinness, 2004).

- *Work environment* – Through conducting focus groups with home health staff nurses and subsequent analysis, Flynn and Deatrick (2003) identified home care agency attributes important to the support of professional practice and job satisfaction. In a subsequent survey of home health nurses, Flynn (2005) identified the ten traits most important to nurses in supporting professional practice. Flynn and colleagues (2005) pooled survey data from home health nurses with an existing data set of hospital-based nurses to determine whether the core set of organizational traits of the nursing practice environment is similarly valued. The program of research on the work environment is still being extended into home health settings (Flynn, 2007).

- *Telehealth* – This is an emerging area of research that is directly linked to home healthcare clinical practice, policy, and administration. While telehealth vendors conduct product research which is limited in scope, others have developed programs of research that advance the science related to the application of telehealth in the home care setting. Current telehealth studies focus on quality of life, impact on patient outcomes, customer satisfaction, safety, and cost comparisons between home visits and the integrative use of telehealth. Some of the early and continuing studies were conducted by Dansky, Palmer, Shea, and Bowles (2001), Dansky, Bowles, and Palmer (1999), and Bowles and Baugh (2007). Their research has focused on the impact of telehealth intervention on patient outcomes. A group of Minnesota researchers investigated the important relationship of telehealth to patient problems, home health nurse interventions, and patient outcomes (Demiris, Speedie, & Finkelstein, 2000; Finkelstein, Speedie, & Potthoff, 2006).

Summary

Because of demographic changes in the population and technological advances, home health nursing continues to be one of the most rapidly growing and changing specialties. Today home health nurses provide skilled care in the home that was not anticipated a few years ago. Home health nurses must be expert in assessment and clinical decision-making skills that form the foundation for home health nursing practice. These skills, combined with a positive attitude and the willingness and ability to adapt to the ever-changing healthcare environment and technology, will help patients and their families and other caregivers to achieve optimal outcomes.

Given the current pandemic warnings and increasing numbers of reports of natural and man-made disasters, home health nurses will experience additional challenges as the home becomes more often the point of care delivery. Home health nurses will be called upon to coordinate and deliver care unlike ever before. The updated scope of practice statement and revised standards of home health nursing practice are meant to guide, define, and direct home health professional nursing practice today as well as in the future.

STANDARDS OF HOME HEALTH NURSING PRACTICE
STANDARDS OF PRACTICE

STANDARD 1. ASSESSMENT
The home health nurse collects comprehensive data pertinent to the patient's health or the situation.

Measurement Criteria:

The home health nurse:

- Collects physical, psychosocial, and environmental data in a systematic, ongoing process.

- Involves the patient, family, and other healthcare providers in holistic data collection.

- Prioritizes data collection activities based on the patient's immediate condition, or anticipated needs of the patient or situation.

- Uses appropriate evidence-based assessment techniques and instruments in collecting pertinent data.

- Uses analytical tools and critical thinking.

- Synthesizes available data, information, and knowledge relevant to the situation to identify patterns and variances.

- Documents relevant data in a retrievable format.

Additional Measurement Criteria for the Advanced Practice Home Health Nurse:

The advanced practice home health nurse:

- Initiates and interprets diagnostic tests and procedures relevant to the patient's current status.

- Conducts comprehensive and in-depth assessments that identify the patient's specialized needs.

STANDARD 2. DIAGNOSIS

The home health nurse analyzes the assessment data to determine the diagnoses or issues.

Measurement Criteria:

The home health nurse:

- Derives the diagnoses and problems based on assessment data.
- Validates the diagnoses or issues with the patient, family, and other healthcare providers.
- Documents diagnoses or issues in a manner that facilitates the determination of the expected outcomes and plan.

Additional Measurement Criteria for the Advanced Practice Home Health Nurse:

The advanced practice home health nurse:

- Compares and contrasts clinical findings with normal and abnormal variations or developmental events systematically in order to formulate a differential diagnosis.
- Uses complex data and information obtained during interview, examination, and diagnostic procedures in identifying diagnoses.
- Assists staff in developing and maintaining competency in the diagnostic process.

STANDARD 3. OUTCOMES IDENTIFICATION
The home health nurse identifies expected outcomes in a plan individualized to the patient and the situation.

Measurement Criteria:

The home health nurse:

- Collaborates with the patient, family, and other healthcare providers in formulating expected outcomes.

- Derives culturally appropriate expected outcomes from the diagnoses.

- Considers associated risks, benefits, costs, current scientific evidence, and clinical expertise when formulating expected outcomes.

- Defines expected outcomes in terms of the patient, patient values, ethical considerations, environment, or situation with such consideration as associated risks, benefits and costs, and current scientific evidence.

- Individualizes expected outcomes in terms of the patient, patient values, ethical considerations, and the environment.

- Includes a time estimate for attainment of expected outcomes.

- Develops expected outcomes that provide direction for continuity of care.

- Modifies expected outcomes based on changes in the status of the patient or evaluation of the situation.

- Documents expected outcomes as measurable goals.

Additional Measurement Criteria for the Advanced Practice Home Health Nurse:

The advanced practice home health nurse:

- Identifies expected outcomes that incorporate scientific evidence and are achievable through implementation of evidence-based practices.

Continued ▶

Standards of Home Health Nursing Practice

- Identifies expected outcomes that incorporate cost and clinical effectiveness, patient satisfaction, and continuity and consistency among providers.

- Uses clinical guidelines that support positive patient outcomes.

- Analyzes the outcome of home health care for specific patient populations to make recommendations for improvement in care delivery systems.

Standard 4. Planning
The home health nurse develops a plan that prescribes strategies and alternatives to attain expected outcomes.

Measurement Criteria:

The home health nurse:

- Develops an individualized plan considering patient beliefs, values, characteristics and the situation (e.g., age- and culturally appropriate, environmentally sensitive).

- Develops the plan in conjunction with the patient, family and other caregivers, members of the interdisciplinary team, and others.

- Includes strategies within the plan that address each of the identified diagnoses or issues, which may include strategies for promotion and restoration of health and prevention of illness, injury, and disease.

- Provides for continuity within the plan.

- Incorporates an implementation pathway or timeline within the plan.

- Establishes the plan to provide direction to others members of the healthcare team.

- Develops the plan to reflect current statutes, rules and regulations, and standards.

- Integrates current trends and research in the planning process.

- Considers the economic impact of the plan.

- Uses standardized language or recognized terminology to document the plan.

Additional Measurement Criteria for the Advanced Practice Home Health Nurse:

The advanced practice home health nurse:

- Identifies strategies that reflect current evidence, research, literature, and expert clinical knowledge.

- Selects or designs strategies to meet the multifaceted needs of complex patients.

STANDARD 5. IMPLEMENTATION
The home health nurse implements the individualized patient plan.

(Implementation includes direct care and coordination of care and teaching.)

Measurement Criteria:

The home health nurse:

- Implements the individualized patient plan in a safe and timely manner.
- Uses evidence-based interventions and treatments.
- Uses the plan to provide direction to other members of the health-care team.
- Documents implementation and changes to the identified plan.

Additional Measurement Criteria for the Advanced Practice Home Health Nurse:

The advanced practice home health nurse:

- Promotes enhanced interdisciplinary and intradisciplinary practice.
- Institutes new evidence-based knowledge and strategies to initiate change in nursing care practices if desired outcomes are not achieved.

STANDARD 5A: COORDINATION OF CARE
The home health nurse coordinates care delivery.

Measurement Criteria:

The home health nurse:

- Coordinates implementation of the plan.

- Facilitates effective uses of resources and systems.

- Uses family, community, financial, and technological resources and systems to implement the plan.

- Collaborates with nursing colleagues and other disciplines to implement the plan.

- Documents the coordination of care.

Measurement Criteria for the Advanced Practice Home Health Nurse:

The advanced practice home health nurse:

- Synthesizes data and information to prescribe necessary system and community support measures, including environmental modifications.

- Provides leadership in the coordination of multidisciplinary healthcare teams for integrated delivery of patient care services.

- Coordinates system and community resources that enhance delivery of care across continuums.

STANDARD 5B: HEALTH TEACHING AND HEALTH PROMOTION
The home health nurse employs strategies to promote health and a safe environment.

Measurement Criteria:

The home health nurse:

- Provides health teaching that addresses such topics as healthy lifestyles, risk-reducing behaviors, home safety, medication management, developmental needs, activities of daily living, and preventive self-care.

- Uses health promotion and health teaching methods appropriate to the situation and the patient's developmental level, learning needs, readiness, ability to learn, language preference, and culture.

- Evaluates the effectiveness of teaching by assessing the patient's learning.

Additional Measurement Criteria for the Advanced Practice Home Health Nurse:

The advanced practice home health nurse:

- Synthesizes empirical evidence on risk behaviors, learning theories, behavioral change theories, motivational theories, epidemiology, and other related theories and frameworks when designing health information and patient education.

- Designs health information and patient education appropriate to the patient's developmental level, learning needs, readiness to learn, and cultural values and beliefs.

- Evaluates health information resources within the area of practice for accuracy, readability, and comprehensibility to help patients access quality health information.

Standard 5c: Consultation

The advanced practice home health nurse provides consultation to influence the identified plan, enhance the abilities of others, and effect change.

Measurement Criteria for the Advanced Practice Home Health Nurse:

The advanced practice home health nurse:

- Synthesizes clinical data, theoretical frameworks, and evidence when providing consultation.

- Facilitates the effectiveness of a consultation by involving the patient and staff in decision-making and negotiating role responsibilities.

- Provides consultation to facilitate organizational change.

STANDARD 5D: PRESCRIPTIVE AUTHORITY AND TREATMENT

The advanced practice home health nurse uses prescriptive authority, procedures, referrals, treatments, and therapies in accordance with state and federal laws and regulations.

Measurement Criteria for the Advanced Practice Home Health Nurse:

The advanced practice home health nurse:

- Prescribes evidence-based treatments, therapies, and procedures considering the patient's comprehensive healthcare needs.

- Prescribes pharmacologic agents based on a current knowledge of pharmacology and physiology.

- Prescribes specific pharmacological agents and treatments based on clinical indicators, the patient's status and needs, and the results of diagnostic and laboratory tests.

- Evaluates therapeutic and potential adverse effects of pharmacological and non-pharmacological treatments.

- Provides patients with information about intended effects and potential adverse effects of proposed prescriptive therapies.

- Provides information about costs and alternative treatments and procedures, as appropriate.

STANDARD 6. EVALUATION
The home health nurse evaluates progress toward attainment of outcomes.

Measurement Criteria:

The home health nurse:

- Conducts a systematic, ongoing evaluation of the patient's outcomes prescribed by the plan and the timeline.
- Includes the patient and others in the evaluative process.
- Evaluates the effectiveness of the planned strategies in relation to patient responses and the attainment of the expected outcomes.
- Uses ongoing assessment data to revise the diagnoses, plan, and implementation strategies as needed to promote optimal patient outcomes.
- Discusses the results with the patient and others involved in the care in accordance with state and federal laws and regulations.
- Documents the results of the evaluation.

Additional Measurement Criteria for the Advanced Practice Home Health Nurse:

The advanced practice home health nurse:

- Evaluates the accuracy of the diagnosis and effectiveness of the interventions in relation to the patient's attainment of expected outcomes.
- Synthesizes the results of the evaluation to determine the impact of the plan on the affected patients, families, groups, communities, and institutions.
- Uses the results of the evaluation to make or recommend process or structural changes including policy, procedure, or protocol documentation.

STANDARDS OF PROFESSIONAL PERFORMANCE

STANDARD 7. QUALITY OF PRACTICE
The home health nurse systematically enhances the quality and effectiveness of nursing practice.

Measurement Criteria:

The home health nurse:

- Demonstrates quality through the application of the nursing process in a responsible, accountable, and ethical manner.

- Uses the results of quality improvement activities to initiate changes in nursing practice and in the healthcare delivery system.

- Incorporates creativity and innovation in nursing practice to improve the quality of care delivery.

- Incorporates evidence-based knowledge into nursing practice to enhance patient outcomes.

- Participates in quality improvement activities. Such activities may include:

  - Identifying aspects of practice important for quality monitoring.

  - Using indicators developed to monitor quality and effectiveness of nursing practice.

  - Collecting data to monitor quality and effectiveness of nursing practice.

  - Analyzing quality indicators and other data to identify opportunities for improving nursing practice and patient outcomes.

  - Formulating recommendations based on quality indicators and other data to improve nursing practice and patient outcomes.

  - Implementing activities based on quality indicators and other data to improve nursing practice and patient outcomes.

  - Analyzing, evaluating, and recommending new technologies to improve patient outcomes.

Continued ▶

- Developing, implementing, and evaluating policies, procedures, and guidelines to improve the quality of nursing practice and patient outcomes.

- Serving as the interdisciplinary team leader or member to evaluate clinical care and health services.

- Determining cost-effective care based on patient need.

- Analyzing factors related to safety, satisfaction, effectiveness, and cost–benefit options.

- Identifying barriers within organizations.

Additional Measurement Criteria for the Advanced Practice Home Health Nurse:

The advanced practice home health nurse:

- Obtains and maintains professional certification if it is available in the area of expertise.

- Designs quality improvement initiatives.

- Implements initiatives to evaluate the need for change.

- Evaluates the practice environment and quality of nursing care rendered in relation to existing evidence, identifying opportunities for the initiation, support, and use of research.

- Analyzes barriers within organizations.

- Implements processes to remove or decrease barriers within organizations.

STANDARD 8. EDUCATION
The home health nurse attains knowledge and competency that reflects current nursing practice.

Measurement Criteria:

The home health nurse:

- Identifies learning needs through self-reflection and inquiry.

- Participates in ongoing educational activities related to appropriate knowledge bases and professional issues.

- Demonstrates a commitment to lifelong learning.

- Seeks experiences that reflect current practice in order to maintain skills and competence in clinical practice or role performance.

- Acquires knowledge and skills appropriate to the specialty area, practice setting, role, or situation.

- Maintains competencies that include interpersonal, technical, and information technology skills.

- Maintains professional records that provide evidence of competency and lifelong learning.

- Seeks experiences and formal and independent learning activities to maintain and develop clinical and professional skills and knowledge.

Additional Measurement Criteria for the Advanced Practice Home Health Nurse:

The advanced practice home health nurse:

- Uses current healthcare research findings and other evidence to expand clinical knowledge, enhance role performance, and increase knowledge of professional issues.

STANDARD 9. PROFESSIONAL PRACTICE EVALUATION

The home health nurse evaluates one's own nursing practice in relation to professional practice standards and guidelines, relevant statutes, rules, and regulations.

Measurement Criteria:

The home health nurse's practice reflects the application of knowledge of current practice standards, guidelines, statutes, rules, and regulations.

The home health nurse:

- Provides age-appropriate care in a culturally and linguistically sensitive manner.

- Engages in self-evaluation of practice on a regular basis, identifying areas of strength as well as areas in which professional development would be beneficial.

- Incorporates feedback from patients, peers, and professional colleagues into professional practice development.

- Participates in systematic peer review as appropriate.

- Takes action to achieve goals identified during the evaluation process.

- Provides rationales for practice beliefs, decisions, and actions as part of the informal and formal evaluation processes.

Additional Measurement Criteria for the Advanced Practice Home Health Nurse:

The advanced practice home health nurse:

- Engages in a formal process seeking feedback regarding one's own practice from patients, peers, professional colleagues, and others.

- Analyzes one's practice in relation to advanced certification requirements.

STANDARD 10. COLLEGIALITY
The home health nurse interacts with peers and colleagues, and contributes to their professional development.

Measurement Criteria:

The home health nurse:

- Shares knowledge and skills with peers and colleagues as evidenced by such activities as patient care conferences or presentations at formal or informal meetings.

- Provides peers and colleagues with feedback regarding their practice or role performance.

- Interacts with peers and colleagues to enhance one's own professional nursing practice or role performance.

- Maintains a supportive relationship with peers and colleagues that increases the effectiveness of the team.

- Contributes to an environment that is conducive to the education of healthcare professionals.

- Contributes to a supportive and healthy work environment.

- Mentors others in home health.

Additional Measurement Criteria for the Advanced Practice Home Health Nurse:

The advanced practice home health nurse:

- Models expert practice to interdisciplinary team members and healthcare consumers.

- Participates in interdisciplinary teams that contribute to role development and advanced nursing practice and health care.

STANDARD 11. COLLABORATION
The home health nurse collaborates with the patient, family, and others in the conduct of nursing practice.

Measurement Criteria:

The home health nurse:

- Communicates with the patient, family, and healthcare providers regarding patient care and the nurse's role in providing that care.

- Collaborates in creating a documented plan focused on outcomes and decisions related to care and delivery of services that indicates communication with patients, families, and others.

- Partners with others to effect change and generate positive outcomes through knowledge of the patient or situation.

- Documents referrals, including provisions for continuity of care.

Additional Measurement Criteria for the Advanced Practice Home Health Nurse:

The advanced practice home health nurse:

- Partners with other disciplines to enhance patient care through interdisciplinary activities and opportunities in education, consultation, management, technological development, or research.

- Facilitates an interdisciplinary process with other members of the healthcare team.

- Documents plan-of-care communications, rationales for plan-of-care changes, and collaborative discussions to improve patient care.

STANDARD 12. ETHICS
The home health nurse integrates ethical principles into all areas of practice.

Measurement Criteria:

The home health nurse:

- Uses *Code of Ethics for Nurses with Interpretive Statements* (ANA, 2001) to guide practice.
- Delivers care in a manner that preserves and protects patient autonomy, dignity, and rights.
- Maintains patient confidentiality within legal and regulatory parameters.
- Serves as a patient advocate assisting patients in developing skills for self advocacy.
- Maintains a therapeutic and professional patient–nurse relationship within appropriate professional role boundaries.
- Contributes to resolving ethical issues of patients, colleagues, or systems as evidenced in such activities as participating on ethics committees.
- Reports illegal, incompetent, or impaired practices.
- Informs the patient of the risks, benefits, and outcomes of healthcare regimens.
- Participates in interdisciplinary teams that address ethical risks, benefits, and outcomes.
- Maintains one's own health and well-being through health-promoting behaviors.

Additional Measurement Criteria for the Advanced Practice Home Health Nurse:

The advanced practice home health nurse:

- Analyzes ethical issues within organizations.
- Participates in interdisciplinary teams that address ethical risks, benefits, and outcomes.

STANDARD 13. RESEARCH
The home health nurse integrates research findings into practice.

Measurement Criteria:

The home health nurse:

- Uses the best available evidence, including research findings, to guide practice decisions.
- Actively participates in research activities at various levels appropriate to the nurse's level of education and position. Such activities may include:
  - Identifying clinical problems specific to nursing research (patient care and nursing practice).
  - Participating in data collection (surveys, pilot projects, formal studies).
  - Participating in a formal committee or program.
  - Sharing research activities and findings with colleagues and others.
  - Conducting research.
  - Using research findings in the development of policies, procedures, and standards of practice in patient care.
  - Incorporating research as a basis for learning.

Additional Measurement Criteria for the Advanced Practice Home Health Nurse:

The advanced practice home health nurse:

- Contributes to nursing knowledge by conducting or synthesizing research that discovers, examines, and evaluates knowledge, theories, criteria, and creative approaches to improve home health practice.
- Formally disseminates research findings through activities such as presentations, publications, consultation, and journal clubs.
- Critically analyzes and interprets research for application to practice.
- Develops evidence-based education programs to improve and standardize the delivery of evidence-based care for the nursing team.

STANDARD 14. RESOURCE UTILIZATION

The home health nurse considers factors related to safety, effectiveness, cost, and impact on practice in the planning and delivery of nursing services.

Measurement Criteria:

The home health nurse:

- Evaluates factors such as safety, effectiveness, availability, cost and benefits, efficiencies, and impact on practice when choosing practice options that would result in the same expected outcome.

- Assists the patient and family in identifying and securing appropriate and available services to address health-related needs.

- Assigns or delegates tasks, based on the needs and condition of the patient, potential for harm, stability of the patient's condition, complexity of the task, and predictability of the outcome.

- Assists the patient and family in becoming informed consumers about the options, costs, risks, and benefits of treatment and care.

- Uses organizational and community resources to formulate interdisciplinary plans of care.

Additional Measurement Criteria for the Advanced Practice Home Health Nurse:

The advanced practice home health nurse:

- Develops innovative solutions for patient care problems that address effective resource utilization and maintenance of quality.

- Develops evaluation strategies to demonstrate cost effectiveness, cost–benefit, and efficiency factors associated with nursing practice.

- Analyzes the outcomes of care related to organizational care delivery for the populations served to make recommendations for improvement in care delivery systems of home healthcare patients.

STANDARD 15. LEADERSHIP

The home health nurse provides leadership in the professional practice setting and the profession.

Measurement Criteria:

The home health nurse:

- Engages in team efforts as a team leader, team builder, and team player.

- Works to create and maintain healthy work environments in local, regional, national, or international communities.

- Displays the ability to define a clear vision, the associated goals, and a plan to implement and measure progress.

- Demonstrates a commitment to lifelong learning for self and others.

- Teaches others to succeed, by mentoring and other supportive strategies.

- Exhibits creativity and flexibility through times of change.

- Demonstrates energy, excitement, and a passion for quality work.

- Willingly accepts mistakes by self and others, thereby creating a culture in which risk-taking is not only safe, but expected.

- Inspires loyalty by valuing people as the most precious asset in an organization.

- Directs the coordination of care across settings and among caregivers, including oversight of licensed and unlicensed personnel in any assigned or delegated tasks.

- Serves in key roles in the work setting by participating in committees, councils, and administrative teams.

- Promotes advancement of the profession through participation in professional organizations.

- Advocates in the political arena for healthcare systems that eliminate health disparities and promote excellent health outcomes for all members of society.

Additional Measurement Criteria for the Advanced Practice Home Health Nurse:
The advanced practice home health nurse:

- Works to influence decision-making bodies to improve patient care.

- Provides direction to enhance the effectiveness of the healthcare team.

- Initiates and revises protocols or guidelines to reflect evidence-based practice, to reflect accepted changes in care management, or to address emerging problems.

- Promotes communication of information and advancement of the profession through writing, publishing, and presentations for professional or lay audiences.

- Designs innovations to effect change in practice and improve health outcomes.

GLOSSARY

Advocacy. Actions intended to maximize patient autonomy and self-determinism through informing, supporting, and affirming a patient's decisions.

Agency/Organization. A formal entity that runs the home care department and that provides home health services to patients of a home health agency or hospital.

Assessment. A systematic, dynamic process by which the registered nurse, through interaction with the patient, significant others, and health-care practitioners, collects and analyzes data about the patient. Data may include the following dimensions: physical, psychological, socio-cultural, spiritual, cognitive, functional abilities, developmental, economic, and life-style.

Care management. An organized system or process for delivering health care to a patient, including assessment, development of a plan of care, initiation and coordination of referrals and services, and evaluation of care. As a care manager, the home health nurse focuses on meeting the comprehensive needs of patients while maximizing appropriate resources and service utilization and acting as a patient advocate.

Caregiver. Anyone who provides care to a patient.

Clinical practice guidelines. Systematic statements designed to help clinicians in making decisions about care. Generally, a group of expert decision-makers are convened to perform a systematic literature review and make specific recommendations based on the evidence.

Complementary and Alternative Medicine (CAM). A group of diverse medical and healthcare systems, practices, and products not presently considered as part of conventional or D.O. (doctor of osteopathy) degrees and by physical therapists, psychologists, and registered nurses. Some healthcare providers practice both CAM and conventional medicine. *Complementary medicine* is used *together with* conventional medicine (e.g., aromatherapy to help lessen a patient's discomfort following surgery). *Alternative medicine* is used *in place of* conventional medicine (e.g., a special diet to treat cancer instead of undergoing surgery, radiation, or chemotherapy).

Cultural therapy. Therapies and treatments used by ethnic, religious, or other cultural groups to promote health and healing. These therapies are usually neither helpful nor harmful from a professional perspective.

Diagnosis. A clinical judgment about the patient's response to actual or potential health conditions or needs. Diagnoses provide the basis for determination of a plan of care to achieve expected outcomes. Registered nurses use nursing or medical diagnoses depending on educational and clinical preparation and legal authority.

Disease management. Coordinated healthcare interventions aimed at specific populations with conditions in which patient self-care efforts are significant, such as heart failure, diabetes, and chronic lung disease.

Electronic health record (EHR). Longitudinal collection of clinical and demographic patient-specific information, stored in a computer-readable format.

Evaluation. The process of determining the progress toward attainment of expected outcomes. Outcomes include the effectiveness of care when addressing one's practice.

Evidence-based practice. A process founded on the collection, interpretation, and integration of valid, important, and applicable patient-reported, clinician-observed, or research-derived evidence. The best available evidence, moderated by patient circumstances and preferences, is applied to improve the quality of clinical judgments.

Family. Family of origin or significant others as identified by the patient.

Home. The patient's residence, which may include a private home or an assisted living or personal care facility.

Home health nursing. A specialized area of nursing practice, rooted in community health nursing, that delivers care in the residence of the patient.

Implementation. Activities such as teaching, monitoring, providing, counseling, delegating, and coordinating.

Information management. Integration of clinical, demographic, financial, administrative, and staffing data; manipulation or processing of these data; and production of various reports that transform data into meaningful information for decision-making.

Interdisciplinary team. A team that includes members from different professions and occupations who work together closely and communicate frequently to optimize care for the patient. Each team member contributes knowledge, skills, and experience to support and augment the contributions of other team members.

Outcomes. Measurable changes in a patient's health status between two or more points in time; in particular, the intervention, intermediate, and end points of nursing and health care.

Plan of care. Comprehensive outline of care to be delivered to attain expected outcomes. It can include prescriptive plans of all disciplines involved with the patient's home health care.

Qualitative data. Pertinent subjective patient-specific narrative details that are derived from interviews, documents, and observation of interactions; the data collector focuses on the whole to give meaning to life experiences.

Quantitative data. Pertinent objective patient-specific numerical details that can be counted and measured consistently; the data collector focuses on the parts to identify positive or negative trends.

Self-management. A patient, family, or caregiver managing an illness or disability independently, keeping the patient as healthy as possible on a daily basis, and identifying early signs of trouble that need additional medical or nursing intervention.

Standard. An authoritative statement defined and promoted by the profession, by which the quality of practice, service, or education can be evaluated.

Standards of care. Authoritative statements that describe a competent level of clinical nursing practice demonstrated through assessment, diagnosis, outcomes identification, planning, implementation, and evaluation.

Standards of nursing practice. Authoritative statements that describe a level of care or performance common to the profession of nursing, by which the quality of nursing practice can be judged. Standards of clinical nursing practice include both standards of care and standards of professional performance.

Standards of professional performance. Authoritative statements that describe a competent level of behavior in the professional role, including quality of practice, education, professional performance evaluation, collegiality, collaboration, ethics, research, resource utilization, and leadership.

REFERENCES

American Nurses Association (ANA). (1999). *Scope and standards of home health nursing practice.* Washington, DC: American Nurses Publishing.

————. (2001). *Code of ethics for nurses with interpretive statements.* Washington, DC: American Nurses Publishing.

————. (2003) *Nursing's social policy statement* (2nd ed.). Washington, DC: Nursesbooks.org.

————. (2004) *Nursing: Scope and standards of practice.* Washington, DC: Nursesbooks.org.

————. (2005) *Recognition of a specialty, approval of scope statements, and acknowledgment of nursing practice standards.* Washington, DC: Nursesbooks.org.

————. (2006). *ANA recognized terminologies and data element sets.* Retrieved September 25, 2007, from http://nursingworld.org/npii/.

Bowles, K.H. (2000). Patient problems and nurse interventions during acute care and discharge planning. *Journal of Cardiovascular Nursing, 14*(3), 29–41.

Bowles, K.H., & Baugh, A.C. (2007). Applying research evidence to optimize telehomecare. *Journal of Cardiovascular Nursing, 22*(1), 5–15.

Brantley, D., Laney-Cummings, K., & Spivack, R. (2004). *Innovation, demand, and investment in telehealth.* U.S. Dept. of Commerce: Office of Technology Policy. Retrieved September 25, 2007 from http://www.technology.gov.reports/TechPolicy/Telehealth/2004Report.pdf.

Brooten, D., Naylor, M.D., York, R., Brown, L.P., Hazard, Munro B., et al. (2002). Lessons learned from testing the quality cost model of advanced practice nursing (APN) transitional care. *Journal of Nursing Scholarship, 34*(4), 369–375.

Brooten, D., Youngblut, J.M., Deatrick, J., Naylor, M., & York, R. (2003). Patient problems, advanced practice nursing (APN) interventions, time and contacts across five patient groups. *Journal of Nursing Scholarship, 35*(1), 73–79.

Centers for Disease Control and Prevention (CDC). (2004). *The burden of chronic diseases and their risk factors: National and state perspectives 2004*. CDC. Retrieved September 25, 2007, from http://www.cdc.gov/nccdphp/burdenbook2004/index.htm.

Clark, J., & Lang, N.M. (1992). Nursing's next advance: An international classification for nursing practice. *International Nursing Review, 39*(4), 109–111, 128.

Dansky, K.H., Bowles, K.H., & Palmer, L. (1999). How telehomecare affects patients. *Caring, XVIII*(8), 10–14.

Dansky, K.H., Palmer, L., Shea, D., & Bowles, K.H. (2001). Cost analysis of telehomecare. *Telemedicine and e-Health, 7*(3), 225–232.

Demiris, G., Speedie, S., & Finkelstein, S. (2000). A questionnaire for the assessment of patients' impressions of the risks and benefits of home telecare. *Telemedicine and e-Health, 6*(5), 278–284.

Feldman, P.H., Murtaugh, C.M., Pezzin, L.E., McDonald, M.V., & Peng, T.R. (2005). Just-in-time evidence-based email "reminders" in home health care: Impact on patient outcomes. *Health Services Research, 40*(3), 849–864.

Feldman, P.H., Peng, T.R., Murtaugh, C.M., Kelleher, C., Donelson, S.M., McCann, M.E., et al. (2004). A randomized intervention to improve heart failure outcomes in community-based home care. *Home Health Care Services Quarterly, 23*(1), 1–23.

Finkelstein, S.M., Speedie, S.M., & Potthoff, S. (2006). Home telehealth improves clinical outcomes at lower cost for home healthcare. *Telemedicine and e-Health, 12*(2), 128–136.

Flynn, L. (2005). The importance of work environment: Evidence-based strategies for enhancing nurse retention. *Home Healthcare Nurse, 23*(6), 366–371.

Flynn, L. (2007). Extending work environment research into home health settings. *Western Journal of Nursing Research, 29*, 200–212.

Flynn, L., Carryer, J., & Budge, C. (2005). Organizational attributes valued by hospital, home care, and district nurses in the United States and New Zealand. *Journal of Nursing Scholarship, 37*(1), 67–72.

Flynn, L., & Deatrick, J.A. (2003). Home care nurses' descriptions of important agency attributes. *Journal of Nursing Scholarship, 35*(4), 385–390.

Harris, M. (2006). We need your input…This is your opportunity to have a voice in the future of your profession. *Home Healthcare Nurse, 24*(3), 133–135.

Humphrey, C.J., & Milone-Nuzzo, P. (1996–1999). *Manual of home care nursing orientation.* Gaithersburg: Aspen.

Humphrey, C.J., & Milone-Nuzzo, P. (2008). *Manual of home care nursing orientation.* Louisville, KY: C.J. Humphrey Associates.

Huston, C.J. (2006). *Professional issues in nursing: Challenges and opportunities.* Philadelphia: Lippincott Williams and Wilkins, pp. 85–98, 256–261.

Jepson, C., McCorkle, R., Adler, D., Nuamah, I., & Lusk, E. (1999). Effects of home care on caregivers' psychological status. *Image: Journal of Nursing Scholarship, 31*(2), 115–120.

Joint Commission International Center for Patient Safety. *2007 National patient safety goals: Home care.* Retrieved September 25, 2007 from http://www.jcipatientsafety.org.

Madigan, E.A. (2001). Comparison of home health care outcomes and service use for patients with wound/skin diagnoses. *Outcomes Management for Nursing Practice, 5*(2), 63–67.

Madigan, E.A., & Fortinsky, R.H. (2004). Inter-rater reliability of the outcomes and assessment information set: Results from the field. *Gerontologist, 44*(5), 689–92.

Madigan, E.A., & Tullai-McGuiness, S. (2004). An examination of the most frequent adverse events in home care agencies. *Home Healthcare Nurse, 22*(4), 256–62.

Madigan, E.A., Tullai-McGuiness, S., & Fortinsky, R.H. (2003). Accuracy in the outcomes and assessment information set (OASIS): Results of a video simulation. *Research in Nursing and Health, 26*(4), 273–283.

Madigan, E.A., & Vanderboom, C. (2005). Home health nursing research priorities. *Applied Nursing Research, 18*(4), 221–225.

Martin, K.S. (2005). *The Omaha System: A key to practice, documentation, and information management* (2nd ed.). St. Louis: Elsevier.

McDonald, M.V., Pezzin, L.E., Feldman, P.H., Murtaugh, C.M., & Peng, T.R. (2005). Can just-in-time evidence-based "reminders" improve pain management among home health care nurses and their patients? *Journal of Pain and Symptom Management, 29*(5), 474–488.

Mebus, K, & Piskor, B. (2005). Participating in the political process. In M. Harris (Ed.), *Handbook of home health care administration* (4th ed.). Sudbury: Jones and Bartlett.

Monsen, K.A., & Kerr, M.J. (2004). Mining quality documentation for golden outcomes. *Home Health Management and Practice, 16*(3), 192–199.

Murtaugh, C.M., Pezzin, L.E., McDonald, M.V., Feldman, P.H., & Peng, T.R. (2005). Just-in-time evidence-based email "reminders" in home health care: Impact on nurse practices. *Health Services Research, 40*(3), 849–864.

National Association for Home Care & Hospice (NAHC). (2004). *Basic statistics about home care.* Washington, DC; NAHC.

National Association for Home Care & Hospice (NAHC). (2006). *Briggs national quality improvement/hospitalization reduction study.* January

2006. Retrieved September 25, 2007 from http://www.nahc.org/ NAHC/CaringComm/eNAHCReport/datacharts/hospredstudy.pdf.

National Association of Clinical Nurse Specialists (NACNS). (2004). *Statement on clinical nurse specialist practice and education*. Harrisburg, PA: NACNS.

Naylor, M.D., Stephens, C., Bowles, K.H., & Bixby, M.B. (2005). Cognitively impaired older adults: From hospital to home. *American Journal of Nursing, 105*(2), 52–61.

Omaha System. (2006). *Overview*. Retrieved September 25, 2007 from http://www.omahasystem.org.

Rogers, E.M. (1995). *Diffusion of innovation* (4th ed.). New York: The Free Press.

Schumacher, K.L. & Marren, J. (2004). Home care nursing for older adults: State of the science. *Nursing Clinics of North America. 39*(3), 443–471.

Stoker, J. (2003). Home care LPN utilization. *Home Healthcare Nurse, 21*(2), 85–89.

U.S. Department of Health and Human Services. (2002). *2001 Report to Congress on telemedicine*. Retrieved September 25, 2007 from http://www.hrsa.gov/telehealth/pubs/report2001.htm.

U.S. Department of Labor, Bureau of Labor Statistics (2006–2007). Occupational Handbook, 2006–07 ed. *Registered Nurses*. Retrieved September 25, 2007 from http://www.bls.gov/oco/ocos083.htm#conditions.

Utterback, K. & Waldo, B. (2005). Matching point of care devices for positive outcomes. *Home Healthcare Nurse, 23*(7), 452–459.

Walke, L.M., Byers, A.L., McCorkle, R., & Fried, T.R. (2006). Symptom assessment in community-dwelling older adults with advanced chronic disease. *Journal of Pain Symptom Management, 31*(1), 31–37.

Wilson, A. (2005). Benchmarking and home health care. In M. Harris (Ed.), *Handbook of home health care administration* (4th ed.) Sudbury: Jones and Bartlett.

World Health Organization (WHO). (2003). *Adherence to long term therapies: Evidence for action*. Retrieved September 25, 2007, from http://www.who.int/chp/knowledge/publications/adherence_report/en/index.html

———. (2007). *International Statistical Classification of Diseases and Related Health Problems, 10th Revision*. Retrieved September 25, 2007, from http://www.who.int/classifications/icd/en/.

BIBLIOGRAPHY

American Nurses Association (ANA). (1999). *Competencies for telehealth technologies in nursing.* Washington, DC: American Nurses Publishing.

American Nurses Association. (2004). *Nurse administrators: Scope and standards of nursing practice.* Washington, DC: Nursesbooks.org.

Buhler-Wilkerson, K. (2001). *No place like home: A history of nursing and home care in the United States.* Baltimore: Johns Hopkins University Press.

Centers for Medicare & Medicaid Services. (2006). *CMS programs and information.* Retrieved September 25, 2007 from http://www.cms.hhs.gov/.

Cherney, E. (2006). New ways to monitor patients at home, as insurers increasingly cover "telemedicine," companies launch way of devices. *The Wall Street Journal,* April 18, p. D1.

Cimino, J.J. (1998). Desiderata for controlled medical vocabularies in the twenty-first century. *Methods of Information in Medicine, 37*(4–5), 394–403.

Dolan, J., Fitzpatrick, M., & Herrmann, E. (1983). *Nursing in society: A historical perspective* (15th ed.). Philadelphia: Saunders.

Dombi, W.A. (Ed.). (2000). *Home care and hospice law: A handbook for executives.* Washington, DC: Caring Publications.

Donahue, M.P. (1996). *Nursing: The finest art* (2nd ed.). St. Louis: Mosby.

Fesler-Brich, D. (2005). Critical thinking and patient outcomes: A review. *Nursing Outlook, 53*(2), 59–65.

Hegyvary, S.T. (2006). A call for papers on evidence-based problems. *Journal of Nursing Scholarship, 38*(1), 1–2.

Kalisch, P.A., & Kalisch, B.J. (1995). *The advance of American nursing* (3rd ed.). Philadelphia: Lippincott.

Lang, N.M. (Ed.). (1995). *Nursing data systems: The emerging framework.* Washington, DC: American Nurses Publishing.

Milone-Nuzzo, P. (2000). Advanced practice nurses in home care are essential. *Home Healthcare Nurse 18*(1), 22–23.

Milone-Nuzzo, P. (2003). Clinical nurse specialists in home care. *Clinical Nurse Specialist, 17*(5), 234–235.

Neal, J.N., & Madigan, E.A. (2001). *Core curriculum for home health care nursing.* Washington, DC: Home Care University, Home Healthcare Nurses Association.

Robert Wood Johnson Foundation. (2002). *Advanced practice nursing: Pioneering practices in palliative care.* Retrieved September 25, 2007 from http://www.promotingexcellence.org/i4a/pages/Index.cfm?pageID=3775.

Schoesslet, M., & Waldo, M. (2006). The first 18 months in practice: A developmental transition model for the newly graduated nurse. *Journal for Nurses in Staff Development, 22*(2), 47–52.

Stoker, J. (2003). Home care LPN utilization. *Home Healthcare Nurse, 21*(2), 85–89.

Stoker, J., & Phillips, B. (2005). Effective support for certain patient populations: One agency's experience. *Home Healthcare Nurse, 23*(11), 696–698.

Struk, C., Peters, D., & Saba, V. (2006). Community health applications. In V. Saba & K.A. McCormick (Eds.), *Essentials of nursing informatics* (pp. 355–382). New York: McGraw Hill Publishing.

Transforming Clinical Data into Critical Outcome Information: How to Survive in the New Data-driven World. (2004). *Home Health Care Management and Practice, 16*(3), special issue.

U.S. Department of Health and Human Services. (2002). HRSA. Bureau of Health Professions. Division of Nursing. *Nurse practitioner primary care competencies in specialty areas: Adult, family, gerontological, pediatric, and women's health.* Retrieved September 25, 2007, from http://www.nonpf.org/finalaug2002.pdf.

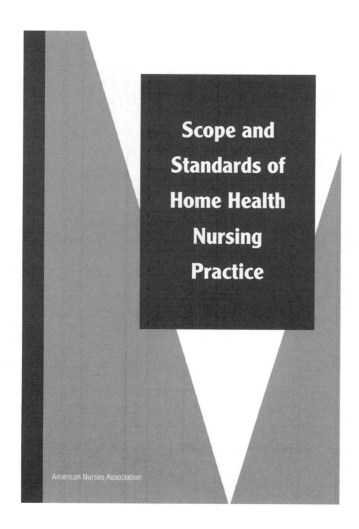

Scope and
Standards of
Home Health
Nursing
Practice

American Nurses Association

SCOPE and STANDARDS
of
Home Health Nursing Practice

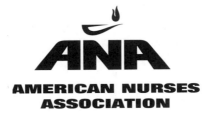

**AMERICAN NURSES
ASSOCIATION**

Library of Congress Cataloging-in-Publication Data

American Nurses Association.
    Scope and standards of home health nursing practice / American
Nurses Association.
        p.   cm.
    Includes bibliographical references.
    1. Home nursing.   2. Visiting nurses.   I. Title.
RT120.H65 A44 1999
610.73'43—dc21

                                                    99-34252
                                                    CIP

Published by
nursesbooks.org
The Publishing Program of ANA
8515 Georgia Avenue
Suite 400
Silver Spring, MD 20910-3492

First printing June 1999. Second printing September 2001. Third printing
December 2002. Fourth Printing June 2005.

9905HH   .5M   06/05R

ACKNOWLEDGMENTS

The task force that created this 1999 revision of the *Scope and Standards of Home Health Nursing Practice* gratefully acknowledges the work of previous task forces, in 1992 and 1986, to initiate the original documents on home health care.

Task Force Members (1999 Scope)

Ann H. Cary, PhD, MPH, RN, ACCC, *Task Force Chair*
Linda M. Sawyer, PhD, RN, CS

The 1999 revision was completed under the auspices of the 1998-2000 ANA Congress of Nursing Practice. The congress gratefully acknowledges the expert review and comments provided by

Emilie Deady, MSN, RN, MGA
Marge Drugay, ND, RN, C
Peggy Galloway, MHSA, BSHCA, RN, CNA
Marilyn D. Harris, MSN, RN, CNAA, FAAN
Margaret Hoffman, BSN, RN, C
Karen Martin, MS, RN, CNAA, FAAN
Karen Schumacher, PhD, RN
Joanne E. Sheldon, MEd, RN, CRNH, CIC

CONTENTS

INTRODUCTION

In 1986, the American Nurses Association first published the *Standards of Home Health Nursing Practice*. These standards were based on the *Standards of Community Health Nursing Practice*, which were revised and published in 1986. Through the development of these two documents, the nursing profession initiated a path of distinction for the home health nurse. In 1992 the *Scope of Practice* document for home health nurses complemented the 1986 standards.

At the dawn of the twenty-first century, this publication, the *Scope and Standards of Home Health Nursing Practice*, provides the template for the performance of professional nurses as well as consumers, payers, and policy makers. Conflicting expectations of nurses in the field of home health care emerge as public policy and reimbursement systems attempt to shape the scope of home health. Consequently, as an example, nurses may be expected to render care that is reimbursable, rather than care that may be necessary or, ultimately, more cost-effective. This revised *Scope and Standards of Home Health Nursing Practice* defines the boundaries of home health nursing practice in the public domain. It acknowledges the changing nature of home health clients, health care delivery financing, and nursing practice, while anchoring the substance of nursing practice in the philosophy of accessibility, affordability, and availability. Recognizing the episodic and intermittent nature of many home health services, this document describes the necessity of practice, which includes the creation of resources through the integration of significant others, and family and community supports; addresses the preventive and health maintenance components of the health-illness trajectory of clients; and endorses the use of evidence-based practice activities.

Historically, the practice of home health evolved in a number of dimensions. In the late 1880s home nursing services were delivered by laypersons who provided nursing care and taught cleanliness and treatment techniques to ill clients and their families. More formal home health services were provided by such nurses as Lillian Wald, who founded public health nursing in 1893 in New York and provided care to the sick poor in their homes. The professional delivery of home health services initiated by visiting nurses and district nurses associations was expanded in the first half of the twentieth century by nurses employed by insurance companies, private free-standing community-based organizations, and a few hospitals. However, with the emergence of funding initiatives for construction and technological development in the hospital setting, the home as a site of care received decreased emphasis until the enactment of the Medicare program in 1965. Since that time, the scope of reimbursable home health services has been broadened by legislation, the number and mix of home care agencies has grown, and more clients have received the benefits of home health nursing care. However, the focus of nursing care in the home has been perplexingly shaped by reimbursement guidelines emphasizing acute, short-term, technologically precise procedures, while at the same time de-emphasizing a comprehensive integration of environmental, social, and caregiver factors into a holistic approach to client care.

During the 1990s the delivery of home health services to clients of all ages has been dramatically influenced by the expansion of managed care systems. As the twenty-first century begins, two additional factors are expected to influence home health practice significantly: prospective payment and outcomes management.

The need for home health services will continue to escalate owing to greater client demand for services, greater public awareness and acceptability of home care, the need for culturally sensitive and linguistically appropriate care, additional reimbursement sources, an increase in the number of elderly clients in the health care system, and adapted technology that allows more services and products to be safely provided in the home care setting. These and other factors will influence the evolution of professional nursing practice in the delivery of home health care through a variety of mechanisms. In the foreseeable future, home health nursing care is likely to be delivered in settings other than a client's residence. Such facilities will likely include community nursing centers; adult day-care programs; group boarding homes; homeless shelters; and intermediate, skilled extended care, and assisted living facilities.

Regardless of the growing trend in demand for home health nursing services, the practice of professional nursing will continue to be grounded in evidence-based clinical knowledge and skills within the framework of family, home, and community concepts. Home health clients need skillful care and the coordination of appropriate community resources to address a variety of needs for these clients, their families, and their supportive caregivers.

SCOPE OF HOME HEALTH NURSING PRACTICE

Definitions and Distinguishing Characteristics

Home health nursing refers to the practice of nursing applied to a client with a health condition in the client's place of residence. Clients and their designated caregivers are the focus of home health nursing practice. The goal of care is to initiate, manage, and evaluate the resources needed to promote the client's optimal level of well-being and function. Nursing activities necessary to achieve this goal may warrant preventive, maintenance, and restorative emphases to prevent potential problems from developing.

Home health nursing is a specialized area of nursing practice with its roots firmly placed in community health nursing. By definition, community health nursing practice includes nursing care directed toward individuals, families, and groups with the predominate responsibility for care being to the population as a whole. The health care needs of the client determine the appropriate augmentation of home health nursing skills with community health nursing practice.

The practice of home health nursing is focused predominately on the care of individuals, in collaboration with the family and designated caregivers. Home health nursing stresses the holistic management of personal health practices for the treatment of diseases or disability. Practice activities embrace primary, secondary, and tertiary prevention; assistance to families; direct care in a client's residence; and coordination of community resources and benefits. Home health nurses assess the biopsychosocial and environmental factors affecting a client's health and support a client-focused nursing care plan addressing a comprehensive approach to the attainment of desired health outcomes. During a client's episode of care, technically precise nursing interventions may be instituted simultaneously with teaching, counseling, care management, resource coordination, and evaluative data collection.

Technical and comprehensive clinical decision-making activities and collaboration in multidisciplinary/interdisciplinary practice further strengthen both the autonomous and interdependent practice demands of home health nursing. The nursing process is the essential vehicle through which goals are achieved.

All nursing care is based on a complete physical, psychosocial, and environmental assessment. In the home setting, the influences of family dynamics and the home environment on the physical and emotional state of the client are essential parameters for care management. The client, family, and caregivers are members of the health care team and will collaborate in the development of the nursing care plans and goals. Because the nurse is a guest in the home, the dynamics of the nurse-client relationship are unique.

In addition, the client's immediate access to other health care resources in the home is limited, so that the nurse's role as a multidisciplinary care coordinator is important in facilitating the goals of care. Because the client often receives services from multiple practitioners and vendors, the home health nurse assumes the role of care manager in coordinating all involved disciplines and directing caregivers to optimize client outcomes. The home health nurse shares knowledge of community health resources with the client's caregivers. This information exchange and advocacy process is used to encourage clients, families, and caregivers to plan for and seek additional services as their needs and resources dictate. Informing, supporting, and affirming client and caregiver decision making is an important adjunct to achieving the nursing care plan and client goals.

The basic conceptualization of home health sets the tone for the nature, allocation, and range of services accessible to clients. Home health care is not merely a change in site or version of acute care delivered at home. Home health requires a change in the definitions and structures of care so that there are a broad array of services and caregivers available to clients experiencing enduring frailty, multidimensional problems, and services outside the realm of normal or standard medical treatment.

Generalist Practice

The professional home health nurse practices at the generalist level in the client's home, site of residence, or appropriate community site. The focus of the nurse's practice includes the client, family, and caregivers. Responsibilities of the generalist include the following.

- Assessing client and caregiver needs.
- Providing client and caregiver education.

- Performing nursing activities within the plan of care.
- Managing resources needed to ensure enactment of the plan of care.
- Providing and monitoring direct and indirect care.
- Collaborating with other disciplines, practitioners, and payers.
- Supervising ancillary personnel and informal caregivers.

The use of the nursing process and advocacy skills are inherent in home health nursing practice. The generalist in home health nursing is prepared at the baccalaureate level.

All professional nurses practicing as home health nurses possess the basic knowledge and skills to carry out the following responsibilities.

- Perform holistic initial and periodic assessments of client and family/caregiver resources to develop and support the plan of care.
- Identify and coordinate community resources and reimbursement resources necessary to support optimal client outcomes.
- Participate in performance improvement activities.
- Collect and use qualitative and quantitative data to evaluate client responses to care; measure outcomes; and monitor the process of care according to the client care plan, reimbursement requirements, and scientific evidence.
- Educate and counsel clients, families, and caregivers to promote self-care activities.
- Initiate health promotion teaching to improve the quality of life, maintain health, and minimize disability.
- Implement the advocacy role through activities that inform, support, and affirm the client and family's self-determination.
- Promote continuity of care through discharge planning, case management, care management, and advocacy.
- Apply the existing body of appropriate evidence-based multidisciplinary knowledge to nursing practice.
- Recognize developmental and biopsychosocial changes in clients, families, and caregivers based on an understanding of psychological, cultural, social, environmental, and spiritual functioning.

- Use the *Scope and Standards of Home Health Nursing Practice,* the appropriate state nursing practice act, and scientific evidence to guide nursing practice.
- Provide direct and indirect care for the client, as appropriate.
- Monitor and support client and caregiver participation in furthering the goals of client care.
- Communicate the plan of care to other practitioners.
- Identify ethical issues and participate with clients, families, and the multidisciplinary staff to explore options and achieve resolutions.

Advanced Practice

The advanced practice nurse in home health care can and may be asked to perform all the functions of a generalist. In addition, the advanced practice nurse possesses substantial clinical experience with individuals, families, and groups; expertise in the process of care management and consultation; and proficiency in planning, implementing, and evaluating programs, resources, services, and research for health care delivery to clients with complex conditions. The specialist in home health nursing is prepared at the graduate level as a clinical nurse specialist and/or a nurse practitioner.

All advanced practice nurses in home health possess advanced nursing knowledge and skills to carry out the following responsibilities.

- Provide consultation to the generalist who is participating in the delivery of care to high-risk home health clients.
- Design, monitor, and evaluate the quality improvement process and risk management components of the clinical program.
- Identify and design research projects based on data generated from the quality improvement program and clinical observations.
- Serve as a resource to the nurse generalist in the identification and evaluation of research findings for application to home health nursing practice.

- Educate the nurse generalist and other health team members about technical, environmental, cognitive, and clinical developments emerging for care of the home health client.
- Perform direct care and document care for select clients and caregivers who require specialist expertise.
- Manage and evaluate the care delivered by caregivers to prevent the reoccurrence of the health care problems in complex cases.
- Design, monitor, and evaluate the client's care management system so that case mix and care demands of clients are met in an optimal manner.
- Monitor and evaluate trends and patterns of reimbursement for home health care.
- Participate in developing and evaluating agency policy and procedures to promote continuity of care from pre-admission to post-discharge activities.
- Facilitate a multidisciplinary and inter-organizational plan of service when barriers to access and utilization are detected.
- Consult with staff and clients on ethical issues related to treatment and self-determinism.
- Supervise an interdisciplinary team and oversee the care management of a population of clients.
- Disseminate practice innovations and research findings to the professional community.

Ethical Considerations for the Home Health Nurse

Owing to the complex nature of home health services and the predominately vulnerable populations home health serves, the ethical issues that arise pose dilemmas that will benefit from identification, discussion, and reflection by all parties. Premature discharge of clients based on expired or diminished reimbursement sources can influence the decision to provide home care. Clients who are underserved and families who are unable to successfully meet the demands of care can pose difficult dilemmas for the health care organization and nurse. Clients, families, and caregivers may demand or need services that are not required or reimbursed by insurance sources, reject reasonable and beneficial treatment and planning activities, refuse to improve environmental conditions essential to the care plan, or avoid reporting abuse or neglect. Many situations in home health involve the autonomous concerns of different parties— the agency and nurse practitioner, the client, the family caregivers, the community, and the third-party payer. Home health nursing practice must include the use of formal and informal ethical structures or committees that can assist in education, counseling, and supporting all concerned in mediating the ethical dilemmas that arise in home health nursing practice. On the health policy level, scarce resources, societal values, and allocation proposals will continue to provide difficult challenges to the practice of home health nursing.

Conclusion

Increasingly, government and employers are choosing managed care systems as the structures through which health care benefits will be offered, with increasing attention being focused on home health nursing practice. For example, many such insurance plans mandate a finite length of stay for hospitalization, thus increasing the necessity for services previously provided in the hospital setting to now be provided at home. However, home health visits are also being limited by payers. As the site of health care, a client's home only sets the stage for the essential structures, processes, and considerations of nursing practice that must be positioned for optimal client outcomes to be realized. Harnessing the intense involvement of family and informal caregivers, as well as community resources, widens the scope of practice for contemporary home health nursing practice. Blending the professional expertise of home health practice with the need to empower clients and caregivers to participate more fully in health care, a home health nursing practice demonstrates congruence with the values of contemporary society. In this environment, nurses must be knowledgeable about the economics and regulation of health care and provide care that enhances quality outcomes and cost-effectiveness.

STANDARDS OF CARE

Standard I. Assessment

The home health nurse collects client health data.

Measurement Criteria

1. Data collection involves the client, family, community, and other health care practitioners, as appropriate.

2. The priority of data collection is determined by the client's immediate condition or needs.

3. Pertinent data are collected using appropriate assessment techniques and valid and reliable instruments.

4. Relevant data are documented in a retrievable form.

5. Integrity of the data is confirmed by multiple sources and used in a confidential manner.

6. The data collection process is systematic, ongoing, and comprehensive to the client's needs and systems' responses.

Standard II. Diagnosis

The home health nurse analyzes the assessment data in determining diagnoses.

Measurement Criteria

1. Diagnoses are derived from the assessment data.

2. Diagnoses are validated with the physician, client, family, and other health care practitioners, when possible and appropriate.

3. Diagnoses are documented in a manner that facilitates the determination of expected outcomes and plan of care.

4. Diagnoses include condition-specific, health promotion, and disease prevention aspects.

Standard III. Outcome Identification

The home health nurse identifies expected outcomes to the client and client's environment.

Measurement Criteria

1. Outcomes are derived from the assessment and diagnoses at two or more points in time.

2. Outcomes are identified as consistent with scientific evidence.

3. Outcomes are mutually formulated with the client, family, physician, and other health care practitioners, when possible and appropriate.

4. Outcomes are culturally appropriate and realistic in relation to the client's present and potential capabilities.

5. Outcomes are attainable in relation to the resources coordinated for the client.

6. Outcomes include a time estimate for attainment.

7. Outcomes provide direction for continuity of care.

8. Outcomes are documented and measurable.

Standard IV. Planning

The home health nurse develops a plan of care that prescribes intervention to attain expected outcomes.

Measurement Criteria

1. The plan is customized for the client (e.g., age-appropriate, culturally sensitive) and the client's condition, needs, and potential.

2. The plan is developed with the client, family, physician, and other health care practitioners, as appropriate.

3. The plan proposes alternatives for continuity of care along the health care continuum.

4. The plan reflects contemporary resources and acknowledges the cost factor of care within the benefit coverage or other resources.

5. The plan reflects evidence-based nursing practice.

6. The plan provides for continuity of care.

7. Priorities for care are established consistent with client and family desires, benefit package, payer desires, and contemporary evidence.

8. The plan is documented.

9. The plan is sensitive to the changing nature of the client's needs.

Standard V. Implementation

The home health nurse implements the interventions identified in the plan of care.

Measurement Criteria

1. Interventions are consistent with the established plan of care.

2. Interventions are implemented in a safe, timely, and appropriate manner.

3. Interventions are documented.

4. Interventions are implemented in accordance with client and caregiver knowledge.

Standard VI. Evaluation

The home health nurse evaluates the client's progress toward attainment of outcomes.

Measurement Criteria

1. Evaluation is systematic, ongoing, and criterion-based.

2. The client, family, and other health care practitioners are involved in the evaluation process, as appropriate.

3. Ongoing assessment data are used to revise diagnoses, expected goals, the plan of care, and interventions as needed.

4. Revisions in diagnoses, expected goals, and the plan of care are documented.

5. The effectiveness of interventions is evaluated in relation to outcomes.

6. The client's responses to interventions are documented.

7. Evaluation activities measure efficiency, effectiveness, costs, and consistency with client needs and developing scientific evidence.

8. The practitioner documents the client outcomes in a manner consistent with reporting requirements.

STANDARDS OF PROFESSIONAL PERFORMANCE

Standard I. Quality of Care

The home health nurse systematically evaluates the quality and effectiveness of nursing practice.

Measurement Criteria

1. The nurse participates in quality improvement activities. Such activities may include the following.
   - Identification of aspects of care important for quality monitoring.
   - Analysis of quality data to identify opportunities for improving care.
   - Development of policies, procedures, and practice guidelines to improve quality of care.
   - Identification of indicators used to monitor quality, appropriateness, costs, and effectiveness of nursing care.
   - Collection of data to monitor quality, appropriateness, and effectiveness of nursing care.
   - Formulation of recommendations to improve nursing practice or client outcomes.
   - Implementation of activities to enhance the quality of nursing practice.
   - Participation on interdisciplinary teams that evaluate clinical practice or health services.

2. The nurse uses the results of quality improvement activities to initiate changes in nursing practice activities.

3. The nurse uses the results of quality improvement activities to initiate changes throughout the health care delivery system, as appropriate.

Standard II. Performance Appraisal

The home health nurse evaluates his or her own nursing practice in relation to professional practice standards, scientific evidence, and relevant statutes and regulations.

Measurement Criteria

1. The nurse engages in performance self-appraisal on a regular basis, identifying areas of strength as well as areas for professional development.

2. The nurse seeks constructive feedback from peers and management regarding his or her own practice.

3. The nurse takes action to achieve goals identified during performance appraisal.

4. The nurse participates in peer review, as appropriate.

5. The nurse's practice reflects knowledge of current professional practice standards, contemporary science, clinical guidelines, laws, and regulations.

Standard III. Education

The home health nurse acquires and maintains current knowledge and competency in nursing practice.

Measurement Criteria

1. The nurse participates in progressive educational activities related to clinical knowledge and professional issues.

2. The nurse obtains experiences that reflect current clinical practice in order to maintain current clinical competence.

3. The nurse acquires knowledge, competencies, and skills appropriate to home health practice.

Standard IV. Collegiality

The home health nurse interacts with and contributes to the professional development of peers and other health care practitioners as colleagues.

Measurement Criteria

1. The nurse shares knowledge and skills with colleagues.

2. The nurse provides peers with constructive feedback regarding their practice.

3. The nurse interacts with colleagues to enhance his or her own professional nursing practice.

4. The nurse contributes to an environment that is conducive to the clinical education of nursing students, other health profession students, and other employees, as appropriate.

5. The nurse contributes to a supportive and healthy work environment.

Standard V. Ethics

The home health nurse's decisions and actions on behalf of clients are determined in an ethical manner.

Measurement Criteria

1. The nurse's practice is guided by the *Code for Nurses with Interpretive Statements.*

2. The nurse maintains and protects client and agency confidentiality within legal and regulatory parameters.

3. The nurse acts as a client advocate to assist clients and families in developing skills so they can care for and advocate for themselves.

4. The nurse delivers care in a nonjudgmental and nondiscriminatory manner that is sensitive to client diversity.

5. The nurse delivers care in a manner that preserves client autonomy, dignity, and rights.

6. The nurse uses available resources to formulate ethical decisions.

7. The nurse reports fraudulent and neglectful care provided by peers, family members, and other health care practitioners or systems.

Standard VI. Collaboration

The home health nurse collaborates with the client, family, and other health care practitioners in providing client care.

Measurement Criteria

1. The nurse communicates with the client, family, and other health care practitioners regarding client care and nursing's role in the provision of care.

2. The nurse collaborates with the physician, client, family, other health care practitioners, and payers in formulating overall goals and the plan of care, making decisions related to care and the delivery of services, and accessing appropriate services.

3. The nurse consults with other health care practitioners regarding client care, as needed.

4. The nurse initiates referrals, including provisions for continuity of care, as needed.

5. The nurse participates on interdisciplinary teams to achieve designated client outcomes.

6. The nurse coordinates resources for client care.

Standard VII. Research

The home health nurse uses research findings in practice.

Measurement Criteria

1. The nurse utilizes best available evidence, preferably research data, to implement the assessment, plan of care, interventions, and evaluation activities.

2. The nurse participates in research activities as appropriate to the nurse's education and position. Such activities may include the following:
   - Identifying clinical problems suitable for nursing research;
   - Participating in data collection;
   - Participating in a unit, organization, or community research committee or program;
   - Sharing research activities with others;
   - Conducting research;
   - Critiquing research for application to practice;
   - Using research findings in the development of policies, procedures, and practice guidelines for client care;
   - Participating on human subject review committees; and
   - Assuring client knowledge of enrollment in research protocols, possible outcomes, and risks.

Standard VIII. Resource Utilization

The home health nurse assists the client or family in becoming informed consumers about the risks, benefits, and cost of planning and delivering client care.

Measurement Criteria

1. The nurse assesses and communicates to the client and family the factors related to safety, effectiveness, availability, and cost when they are choosing between two or more practice options that would result in the same expected client outcome.

2. The nurse assists the client and family in identifying and securing appropriate and available services to address health-related needs.

3. The nurse assigns or delegates tasks as defined by the state nurse practice acts and according to the knowledge, skills, availability, and willingness of the designated caregiver.

4. If the nurse assigns or delegates tasks, it is based on the needs and condition of the client, the potential for harm, the stability of the client's condition, the complexity of the task, the predictability of the outcome, and the legal implications.

5. The nurse uses appropriate agency and community resources to ensure personal safety.

GLOSSARY

Activities of daily living—Basic activities that a person performs on a daily basis, such as bathing, dressing, eating, toileting, grooming, transferring activities, ambulation/locomotion. Many home health care clients require assistance with such activities.

Advocacy—A role in practice that attempts to maximize client autonomy and self-determinism through informing, supporting, and affirming client decisions.

Assessment—A systematic, dynamic process by which the nurse, through interaction with the client, significant others, and health care practitioners, collects and analyzes data about the client. Data may be collected on the following dimensions: physical, psychological, sociocultural, spiritual, cognitive, functional abilities, developmental, economic, and life-style.

Caregiver—Anyone who provides services to a client.

Care coordination/management—An organized system or process for delivering health care to a client or group of clients, including assessment, development of a plan of care, initiation and coordination of referrals and services, and evaluation care.

Care coordinator—The producer of care coordination and care management.

Client—An individual or family who receives care or services as sanctioned by state nursing practice acts. When the client is an individual, the focus is on the health state, problems, or needs of a single person. When the client is a family or group, the focus is on the health state of the unit as a whole or the reciprocal effects of an individual's health state on the other members of the unit. When the client is a community, the focus is on personal and environmental health and the health risks of population groups.

Community Health Nursing—A synthesis of nursing practice and public health practice applied to promoting and preserving the health of populations. Health promotion; health maintenance; health education; and management, coordination, and continuity of care are used in a holistic approach to the management of the health care of individuals, families, and groups in a community.

Continuity of care—An interdisciplinary process that includes clients and significant others in the development of a coordinated plan of care. This process facilitates the client's transition between settings, based on changing needs and available resources.

Criteria—Relevant, measurable indicators of the standards of clinical nursing practice.

Diagnosis—A clinical judgment about the client's response to actual or potential health conditions or needs. Diagnoses provide the basis for determination of a plan of care to achieve expected outcomes.

Direct care—Care activities that include assessment, diagnosis, outcomes identification, planning, implementation, and evaluation.

Evaluation—The process of determining both the client's progress toward the attainment of expected outcomes and the effectiveness of nursing care.

Evidence-based practice—Nursing practice based on scientific evidence, which establishes a link between practice and outcomes of client care.

Family—The family of origin or significant others, as identified by the client.

Formal caregiver—A caregiver who is paid directly by the client, family, or guardian, or who is employed by a home health care organization.

Guidelines—Descriptions of a process of client care management that has the potential to improve the quality of clinical and consumer decision making. Guidelines are systematically developed statements based on available scientific evidence and expert opinion.

Health care practitioners—Individuals with special expertise who provide health care services or assistance to clients. They may include nurses, physicians, psychologists, social workers, nutritionists/dieticians, pharmacists, various therapists, and aides.

Home health—The range of health care services provided to a client in his or her home or place of residence.

Home health nursing—A specialized area of nursing practice with its roots firmly placed in community health nursing. Nursing care is delivered in the residence of the client.

Implementation—To ensure practical fulfillment of goals by specific measures, including any or all of these activities: intervening, delegating, coordinating. The client, significant others, or health care practitioners may be designated to implement interventions within the plan of care.

Indirect care—Care activities provided on behalf of the client including case management, coordination of resources, and consultation with other health practitioners.

Informal caregiver—A family member, significant other, friend, neighbor, or volunteer who provides services to a client during an episode of illness.

Instrumental activities of daily living—Activities such as shopping, meal preparation, transportation, financial management, homemaking, home maintenance, and the ability to use the phone. These activities are known to maintain a client's independence.

Nurse—Individual who is licensed by a state agency to practice as a registered nurse.

Nursing—The diagnosis and treatment of human responses to actual or potential health problems.

Outcomes—Measurable changes in client health status between two or more points in time; the utilization, intermediate, and end point results of nursing and health care that are measurable.

Plan of care—Comprehensive outline of care to be delivered to attain expected outcomes. It can include prescriptive plans of all disciplines involved with the client's home health care.

Primary prevention—Measures that actively promote health, prevent illness, and provide specific protection.

Professional care—Home health services in which the boundaries of practice are determined by professional standards with a basis in scientific theory and research.

Quality of care—The degree to which health services for individuals and populations increase the likelihood of desired health outcomes consistent with current scientific and professional knowledge.

Quality improvement—A conceptual framework for evaluating the quality of care that emphasizes an analytical approach to understanding the contributions of all components of the health care system in achieving results and constantly incorporating improvements into the system.

Recipients of nursing care—Individuals, groups, families, communities, or a population as a client of care.

Secondary prevention—The early diagnosis measures and prompt interventions aimed at limiting disabilities.

Standard—An authoritative statement enunciated and promulgated by the profession by which the quality of practice, service, or education can be judged.

Standards of care—Authoritative statements that describe a competent level of clinical nursing practice demonstrated through assessment, diagnosis, outcome identification, planning, implementation, and evaluation.

Standards of nursing practice—Authoritative statements that describe a level of care or performance common to the profession of nursing by which the quality of nursing practice can be judged. Standards of clinical nursing practice include both standards of care and standards of professional performance.

Standards of professional performance—Authoritative statements that describe a competent level of behavior in the professional role, including activities related to quality of care, performance appraisal, education, collegiality, ethics, collaboration, research, and resource utilization.

Tertiary prevention—Rehabilitation activities and measures that reduce impairments and disabilities, minimize suffering caused by departures from good health, and promote the client's adjustment to immediate conditions.

BIBLIOGRAPHY

American Nurses Association. *A Conceptual Model of Community Health Nursing*. Kansas City, Mo.: American Nurses Association, 1980, p. 2.

American Nurses Association. *Code for Nurses with Interpretive Statements*. Washington, DC: American Nurses Association, 1985.

American Nurses Association. *Nursing's Social Policy Statement*. Washington, DC: American Nurses Association, 1995.

American Nurses Association. *Scope and Standards of Advanced Practice Registered Nursing*. Washington, DC: American Nurses Association, 1996.

American Nurses Association. *Scope of Practice for Home Health Nursing*. Kansas City, Mo.: American Nurses Association, 1992.

American Nurses Association. *Standards of Clinical Nursing Practice*, 2nd ed. Washington, DC: American Nurses Association, 1998.

American Nurses Association. *Standards of Community Health Nursing Practice*. Kansas City, Mo.: American Nurses Association, 1986.

American Nurses Association. *Standards of Home Health Nursing Practice*. Kansas City, Mo.: American Nurses Association, 1986.

American Nurses Association. *Standards of Nursing Practice*. Washington, DC: American Nurses Association, 1973.

Beuscher, T. C. The Clinical Nurse Specialist: A Valuable Resource in Home Care. *Caring* 10, no. 4 (1991): 22–25.

Cary, A. H. "Advocacy and Allocation." *Nursing Connections* II, no. I (1998): 35–40.

Cary, A. H. "Case Management." In *Community Health Nursing: Promoting the Health of Aggregates, Families and Individuals*, 5th ed, edited by M. Stanhope and J. Lancaster. St. Louis: Mosby Yearbook, forthcoming.

Cary, A. H. "Institutional Review Boards and Bioethics Committees: Their Role in Ensuring Ethical Home Care Research." *Home Care Economics* 1, no. 4 (1987): 113–118.

Collopy, B., Dubler, N., and Zuckerman, C. "The Ethics of Home Health Care: Autonomy and Accommodation," *The Hastings Center Report* 20, no. 2 (1990): 3 (supplement).

Deming, W. E. *Out of Crisis*. Cambridge: Massachusetts Institute of Technology, 1982.

Duffus, R. L. *Lillian Wald: Neighbor and Crusader*. New York: Macmillan, 1938, pp. 23–26.

Green, J. L., and Driggers, B. "All Visiting Nurses Are Not Alike: Home Health and Community Health Nursing." *Journal of Community Health Nursing* 6, no. 2 (1989): 83–93.

Hanlon, J. J. *Public Health Administration and Practice*, 6th ed. St. Louis: Mosby, 1979, pp. 654–656.

Henderson, V. *Basic Principles of Nursing Care*. London: International Council of Nurses, 1961, p. 42.

Humphrey, C. J. "The Home as a Setting for Care: Clarifying the Boundaries of Practice." *Nursing Clinics of North America* 22, no. 1 (1988): 305–314.

Humphrey, C. J., and Nuzzo, P. M. *Manual of Home Care Nursing Orientation*. Gaithersburg, Md.: Aspen, 1999.

Reider, A. "Potential Liability for Institutional Review Boards and Bioethics Committee." *Home Care Economics* 1, no. 4 (1987): 119–121.

Reif, L. J., and Martin, K. S. *Nurses and Consumers: Partners in Assuring Quality Care in the Home.* Washington, DC: American Nurses Association, 1995.

Sawyer, L. M. "Community Health Nurse in Home Health and Hospice." In *Community Health Nursing: Promoting the Health of Aggregates, Families and Individuals,* 5th ed., edited by M. Stanhope and J. Lancaster. St. Louis: Mosby Yearbook, forthcoming.

Shaughnessy, P. W. and Crisler, K. S. *Outcomes-Based Quality Improvement.* Denver: Colorado Center for Health Policy and Services Research, 1995.

U.S. Department of Health and Human Services. *Federal Register,* Part II, CFR Parts 484 and 488 (Jan. 25, 1999), p. 42.

Warhola, C. F. *Planning for Home Health Services: A Resource Hand-Book.* U.S. Department of Health and Human Services, Washington, DC, 1980.

INDEX

Pages in the 1999 *Scope and Standards of Home Health Nursing Practice* are marked by square brackets, e.g., [71, 73].

A
ABC Codes, 21
Accountability, *vii*, 17
  quality of practice and, 41
Activities of daily living (defined), [88]
Acute care, 1, 2, 10, [71, 73]
  patient education, 12
  pharmacologic treatment, 9
  research, 25
  safety, 16
  See also Hospitalization
Administration, 10, 14, 23, 26
Advanced practice home health
    nursing, 9–10, 25, [75–76]
  assessment, 29, [78]
  collaboration, 46, [85]
  collegiality, 45, [84]
  consultation, 37
  coordination of care, 35
  diagnosis, 30, [78]
  education, 43, [83]
  ethics, 47, [84–85]
  evaluation, 39, [80–81]
  health teaching and health promotion,
    36
  implementation, 34, [80]
  leadership, 50–51
  outcomes identification, 31–32, [79]
  planning, 33, [79–80]
  prescriptive authority and treatment,
    38
  professional practice evaluation, 44,
    [83]
  quality of practice, 41–42, [82]
  research, 48, [86]
  resource utilization, 49, [86–87]
  roles, 9–15
  See also Home health nursing;
    Generalist practice home health
    nursing

Advanced Practice Registered Nurse
  (APRN), 9
Advocacy, 10, 12, 18, [73, 74]
  defined, 53, [88]
  ethics and, 47, [84]
  generalist practice, [74]
  implementation and, 6
  leadership and, 50
Age-appropriate care, 17, 44
  See also Cultural competence
Agency (defined), 53
American College of Cardiology, 26
American Heart Association, 26
American Nurses Association (ANA), *vii*,
  viii, 1, 26
  Code of Ethics for Nurses with Interpre-
    tive Statements, *vii*, 18, 47, [84]
  Nursing: Scope and Standards of
    Practice, *vii*, 8
  Nursing's Social Policy Statement, *vii*
Analysis. *See* Critical thinking, analysis,
  and synthesis
Assessment, 4, 10, 11, 28, [73]
  defined, 53, [88]
  diagnosis and, 5, 30, [78]
  evaluation and, 39, [81]
  generalist practice, [74]
  implementation and, 6
  outcomes identification and, [79]
  research and, [86]
  standard of practice, 29, [78]
  step in nursing process, *vii*, 4–5
Autonomous practice, 8, 9, 10, 47, [72]

B
Behavioral health, 16
Bertillon, Jacques, 21
Best practice, 10, 18, 25, 26
Body of knowledge, 8, 9, 13, 19, [75]
  education and, 43, [83]

97

Body of knowledge (*continued*)
outcomes identification and, 31
planning and, 33
prescriptive authority and treatment,
38
Breckinridge, Mary, 1

C

Care recipient. *See* Patient
Care standards. *See* Standards of practice
Caregivers, 4
defined, 53, [88]
formal, (defined), [90]
Care management, 8, 9, 10, 11–12, [72]
advanced practice, [75, 76]
defined, 53, [88]
diagnosis and, 5
generalist practice, [74]
hospitalization and, 16
implementation and, 6
planning and, 5
See also Coordination of care
Centers for Medicare and Medicaid
Services (CMS), 18, 22, 25
Certification and credentialing, 7, 14,
19–20
leadership and, 50
planning and, 6
professional practice evaluation and,
42
quality of practice and, 42
standardized nomenclature and, 22
Chronic illness, 10, 12, 15–16, 17
Client. *See* Patient
Clinical concerns in home health
nursing, 15–17
Clinical manager. *See* Supervision
Clinical Nurse Specialist (CNS), 9–10,
[75]
Clinical settings. *See* Practice settings
Code of Ethics for Nurses with
Interpretive Statements, *vii*, 18, 47,
[84]
See also Ethics
Collaboration, 4, 13, 15, [72]
advanced practice, 9, 10

care management, 11, 12
coordination of care and, 35
diagnosis and, 5
generalist practice, [74]
implementation and, 6
outcomes identification and, 31
planning and, 5
standard of professional performance,
46, [85]
research and, 26, 27
See also Healthcare providers;
Interdisciplinary health care
Collegiality,
ethics and, 47
professional practice evaluation and,
44, [83]
standard of professional performance,
45, [84]
Communication, 4, 8, [73]
advanced practice, [76]
advocacy and, 13
care management and, 11
collaboration and, 46
collegiality and, 45, [84]
education and, 12
generalist practice, 8, [75]
leadership and, 51
research and, 48, [86]
supervision and, 15
telehealth and, 24
Community health, 3, 12, 17, 27, [71]
evaluation and, 39
Community health nursing (defined), [89]
Community resources, 3, 13, [72, 77]
advanced practice, 9
coordination of care and, 35, [73]
generalist practice, [74]
implementation and, 6
See also Resource utilization
Competence assessment. *See*
Certification and credentialing
Complementary and alternative
medicine, 6
defined, 53
Confidentiality, 17, 18, 47, [78, 84]
See also Ethics

Data collection (*continued*)
  quality of practice and, [82]
  research and, 48, [86]
Decision-making, 4, 14, 28, [72, 73]
  advocacy and, 13
  collaboration and, 46, [85]
  consultation and, 37
  generalist practice, 8
  implementation and, 6
  leadership and, 51
  professional practice evaluation and, 44
  research and, 48
Demographics, 15, 17, 25, 28
Diagnosis, 10, 22
  assessment and, 29
  defined, 54, [89]
  evaluation and, 39, [81]
  outcomes identification and, 5, [79]
  planning and, 33
  prescriptive authority and treatment, 38
  standard of care, 30, [78]
  step in nursing process, *vii*, 5
Diagnosis-related groups (DRGs), 2
Direct care, 11, 24, 34
  defined, [89]
District nurse, 1
Dock, Lavinia, 1
Documentation, 11, 14, 20, 23, [76]
  assessment and, 29, [78]
  collaboration and, 46
  coordination of care and, 35
  diagnosis and, 30, [78]
  education and, 43
  evaluation and, 39, [81]
  implementation and, 34, [80]
  outcomes identification and, 31, [79]
  planning and, [80]

E
Economic issues. *See* Cost control
Education of home health nurses, 7, 11, 12, 13
  advanced practice, 9, 10, [75, 76]
  collaboration and, 46
  collegiality and, [84]

diagnosis and, 30
  generalist practice, 8, [74]
  leadership and, 50
  quality improvement and, 15
  research and, [86]
  standard of professional performance, 43, [83]
  supervision and, 14
  See also Mentoring; Professional development
Education of patients and families, 12, 24, 25, [72, 73]
  care management, 11
  consumerism and, 17
  ethics and, [77]
  generalist practice, [74]
  hospitalization and, 16
  implementation and, 6
  prescriptive authority and treatment, 38
  See also Family; Health teaching and health promotion; Patient
Electronic health record, 23, 24
  defined, 54
End-of-life care, 3, 26
Environmental assessment, 5
Environmental factors, [72, 73]
  See also Practice environment
Ethics, 17–18, [75, 76–77]
  outcomes identification and, 31
  quality of practice and, 41
  research and, [86]
  standard of professional performance, 47, [84–85]
  See also Code of Ethics for Nurses with Interpretive Statements; Laws, statutes, and regulations
Evaluation, 9, 11, 14, [75]
  defined, 54, [89]
  quality of practice and, 42
  research and, [86]
  standard of practice, 39, [80–81]
  step in nursing process, *vii*, 7
Evidence-based practice, 13, 15, 17, [70, 71]
  advanced practice, 9, 10
  assessment and, 29

Internet, 22, 23, 25
Interventions, 3, 4, 9, 10, 13
   evaluation and, 39, [81]
   implementation and, 6, 34, [80]
   research and, 25, [86]
   telehealth and, 24

K
Knowledge base. *See* Body of knowledge

L
Laws, statutes, and regulations, 9, 13,
   14, 18–19, [77]
   ethics and, 47, [84]
   evaluation and, 39
   generalist practice, [75]
   implementation and, 6, 7
   OASIS and, 27
   planning and, 5–6, 33
   prescriptive authority and treatment,
   38
   professional practice evaluation and,
   44, [83]
   resource utilization and, [87]
   See also Ethics
Leadership, 13, 14, [75]
   coordination of care and, 35
   resource utilization and, [87]
   standard of professional performance,
   50–51
   See also Mentoring
Licensed Practical/Vocational Nurse
   (LPN/LVN), 5, 6, 7, 11
Licensing. *See* Certification and
   credentialing
LOINC data standard, 21–22, 24–25
Long-term care, 17

M
Measurement criteria. *See* Criteria
Medicare, 2, 15, 23, [71]
   OASIS and, 22
   planning and, 5
Mentoring, 7, 8, 9, 13, 15
   collegiality and, 45
   leadership and, 50
   See also Education of home health

nurses; Leadership; Professional
   development
Metropolitan Life Insurance Company,
   1
Multidisciplinary healthcare. *See* Interdisciplinary health care

N
National Association for Home Care
   and Hospice (NAHC), *viii*, 2
National Coordinator for Health
   Information Technology, 24
National League for Nursing (NLN), 1–2
Nightingale, Florence, 1, 21
North American Nursing Diagnosis
   Association (NANDA), 21
Nurse (defined), [90]
Nurse Practitioner (NP), 9, 10, [75]
Nursing (defined), [91]
Nursing care standards. *See* Standards
   of care
Nursing Interventions Classification (NIC),
   21
Nursing data sets, 21
Nursing Outcomes Classification (NOC),
   21
Nursing process, *vii*, 4–7, 8, 11, [74]
   quality of practice and, 41
   See also Standards of Practice
Nursing role specialty, 10–15
Nursing shortage, 20
Nursing standards. *See* Standards of
   practice; Standards of professional
   performance

O
Omaha System, 21, 26
Outcome Assessment and Information
   Set (OASIS), 17, 22, 27
Outcomes, 8, 9, 10, 11, 16, [72, 77]
   assessment and, 4
   collaboration and, 46, [85]
   defined, 55, [91]
   diagnosis and, 30, [78]
   ethics and, 47
   evaluation and, 7, 39, [80]
   implementation and, 6, 34

Roles in home health nursing practice (*continued*)

Terminology, 53–56, [88–92]
    planning and, 33
    standardization, 20–22
Tertiary prevention (defined), [92]
Transitional care, 26
Trends in home health nursing practice,
    15, [77]

V
Visiting Nurse Associations (VNAs), 1, [70]

Visiting Nurse Associations of America
    (VNAA), 2
Visiting Nurse Service (VNS), 26–27

W
Wald, Lillian, 1, [70]
Work environment. *See* Practice
    environment
World Health Organization (WHO), 16,
    21

DATE DUE			